CRASH COURSE

on
Losing Weight

21
PRACTICAL
WAYS TO
LOOK
AND FEEL
BETTER

A Division of Thomas Nelson Publishers
Since 1798

www.thomasnelson.com

Copyright © 2006 by Mark Gilroy Communications,
Franklin, Tennessee

Published by J. Countryman® a division of Thomas Nelson, Inc.,
Nashville, Tennessee 37214

Written by Max and Alanna Davis

www.jcountryman.com
www.thomasnelson.com

Designed by Randall Miller Design, Tulsa, Oklahoma

ISBN 1-4041-8654-9

Printed in China

CRASH COURSE

on
Losing Weight

21
PRACTICAL
WAYS TO
LOOK
AND FEEL
BETTER

Table of Contents

Introduction

To the Reader:

You may be thinking, Oh no, not another book on weight loss! How could it possibly be that there would be any need for more information on losing weight? I mean, you can't even go through a grocery check out without seeing headlines of how you can now lose thirty pounds in three days if you will only buy the secrets contained in the magazine. Amazingly, the next time you go to buy groceries, there are new magazines with new secrets!

Well, you won't find any secrets in this Crash Course book on weight loss. What you will find is the tried and tested information you need to know so you can look and feel better. There are no claims in it that you can easily shed pounds and get physically fit without effort. No, that is the stuff of fantasy and we leave it to be hawked at the grocery checkouts.

If you are ready to make the needed changes in you life to once and for all win the weight loss fight, than you have found the right book. The authors, Max and Alanna Davis, lay it all on the line, plain and simple.

They tell you that in order to get fit you will have to change your thinking—and then they lead you through the steps to do so. This is really important information. We all know that until habits change, weight loss will always remain a struggle. And in order to change habits, it is necessary to change your thinking. But how do you do that? You will find out exactly how to do so in the first several chapters.

Then throughout the book you will find the information you need on what habits lead to weight gain and which to weight loss. You will also get the low down on what you will need to do to get your body moving again and in shape—just the way you want it to be.

I think you will really be intrigued, as I was, on the depth and breadth of the information provided in this book. Best of all, this information is laid out by the authors in an interesting way with real life examples from people who have used the principles listed in this book to achieve their fitness goals. In the following pages, look for practical hints and Success in Their Own Words segments based on interviews done by the authors. Yeah, it's a Crash Course, but it's got all of the factual information everyone needs to shed pounds.

So go for it! Dare to become one of the 36% of Americans who are not overweight!

Good Luck,

Larry J. Koenig, Ph.D.
General Editor and Series Consultant

Making the Connection

All of us have the ability to become wonderfully stronger—physically, mentally, emotionally and spiritually—no matter where we are on the health continuum. All of us can achieve a new level of fitness at any point in our lives if we understand how we are connected: body, mind, and spirit.

—TERRY DORIAN, PH.D.

POWER STATEMENT:

> Losing weight starts with changing the way we think about ourselves, food, and exercise.

At age forty-four, Kathy Manning looks and feels incredible. In fact, she actually looks and feels better today than she did in high school. Those who have only known her for a short period of time find it difficult to believe that Kathy was once overweight, unhealthy, and depressed. What else is so incredible about her story is that Kathy has maintained her transformation for over seventeen years now and has little fear of ever reverting back to her former self. She is living proof that long-term transformations are not merely pie-in-the-sky dreams, but are actually attainable.

Throughout her teen years, Kathy had been fairly active. For three years, she danced on the school's dance team, a group that performed with the band during halftimes at football and basketball games. Dancing kept her burning the calories. In the later part of her senior year, however, after the last season of dance had finished, Kathy began to suddenly gain weight, and for the next decade, she found herself locked in a frustrating struggle to lose it.

She tried one fad diet after the other, yet regardless of what she did or how hard she worked, nothing gave her the lasting results she wanted. The more she tried, the harder the rebound effect would hit her. Once, she attempted a "starvation diet" in which she would skip meals, but then would wind up overeating later on. About the only consistent thing she did take away from all the dieting was poor eating habits. Kathy had even led an aerobics class at her church, but despite all her efforts, ten years after high school she'd added on another thirty pounds and was a very unhealthy and unhappy person.

In an interview, Kathy told me the day that will go down in her life as a major turning point was the day she discovered she was pregnant with her now sixteen-year-old daughter. "I wanted to be fit for my baby and have a healthy pregnancy. I also knew that if I stayed on my present course, I would only get heavier after the baby was born. I was desperate."

With new motivation coming from the baby growing inside her womb, Kathy set out to learn everything she could, not just about losing weight, but being a healthy person. The education she received helped catapult her into long-term weight loss and into a whole new lifestyle of being active and feeling better about herself.

The first step to that lasting change happened when she made the connection between her thinking patterns and her health. Before she could have the results she desired, she had to change the way she thought about herself, food, exercise, and healthy living in general. She came to understand that part of her weight problems were linked to deep-seated emotional issues. Because of poor self-esteem, she often found herself eating for comfort. Another reason she ate was simply because the food was there, and for recreation. It seemed whenever she went out or got together with friends and family, all they did was eat.

Kathy told me she began to see results when she started seeing food as a "sustainer instead of a comforter." Though it didn't happen all at once, she stopped eating simply to eat and trained herself to think differently about food. Because she now saw food as her sustainer, it became easier to eat things that contributed to good health rather than rob her of good health. She paid close attention to what she put into her body. Kathy said, "Instead of thinking about how much I could get away with eating, I started thinking about how much I could get away with not eating. I started eating smaller portions. If I ate something sweet, I would just eat a very small bit." To Kathy's surprise, what she discovered was that she could eat healthy, be satisfied, and still enjoy food. Instead of having to diet to lose weight, when she ate healthy, the weight came off naturally.

In addition to changing the way she thought about food, she began a regular sustained exercise program. "It just became a part of who I was. Just like I took a bath and brushed my teeth, I would come home from work, put on my sneakers, and go walking. After I had the baby, I simply kept it up."

Then, somewhere along Kathy's journey to fitness and health, she began to think differently not just about food and exercise, but about herself. Little by little, she felt better about who she was and how she looked. As her energy level increased, so did her self-esteem. "In the past, I hated myself and felt imprisoned in a body and life that I could do nothing about, but then I started seeing myself as free to be thin and seeing all the possibilities I had. We don't have to believe the lies we tell ourselves or that others tell us—God will give us the power to change."

Kathy's story is what this book is all about. It's about 1) making the connection between the way you think about food, exercise, and your health in general, and 2) engaging the power to change your old habits into healthy ones based on your new mindset.

PRACTICAL TIP #1

On an index card, write down why you want to lose weight or revamp your diet and exercise routine. Post it on your bathroom mirror or anywhere else you'll see it frequently. This will serve as a motivator for the journey ahead.

If you're reading this book, you're probably wanting to shed those unwanted pounds and look and feel better. The good news is, although this will require a change in lifestyle instead of an overnight cure, you really do have the ability to help yourself and you won't have to turn your whole life upside down to do it. Regardless of your age, current weight, or particular place you are in life, when it comes to creating a healthier, fitter you, you don't have to settle for less. Like Kathy, along with countless others, you too can make the choice to be the best you that you can be—to look and feel better and fulfill all your potential. By following the proven principles set forth in this book, your life can literally be transformed—not just your weight and figure, but your self-confidence, and you'll stand a better chance at living a longer, richer life. Are you ready to make the change?

PERSONAL REFLECTION:

How long have you battled your weight? Why do you think it's an issue for you?

What do you most want to change about your life? How do you think changing your diet and exercise routines will help you do that?

YOUR TO DO LIST:

Take a walk around the neighborhood. As you walk, use the time to think about your lifestyle and what new habits you might need to develop.

FOR FURTHER STUDY:

Emotional Eating: A Practical Guide to Taking Control
    —by Edward E. Abramson

America, We Have a Problem

Food should be one of life's greatest pleasures. But in today's sound-bite society we have come to focus more on what we shouldn't be eating than on what we should.

—DR. ED BLONZ

POWER STATEMENT:

To create a healthy lifestyle, we have to resist the cultural temptation to neglect exercise and eat convenient, but unhealthy foods.

A ccording to the American Dietetic Association, there are more overweight people in America today than ever before. The Centers for Disease Control and Prevention report that 64% of the U.S. population is overweight or "obese." This shouldn't be too surprising, given the sedentary lifestyle and diet of fast food, junk food, and processed food that our modern culture fosters. Even our household pets are affected. Garfield the cat is more the norm than one might think—according to the National Research Council, 25% of dogs and cats are overweight.

As a society, we are fatter than ever before, mainly because we eat more than ever before and we dine out more than ever before. On top of that, many restaurants pride themselves on serving large portions. Every time we turn around, we are bombarded with mouth-watering food advertisements playing to our cravings, touting their large portions as a bargain. This may be good for your pocketbook, but it's bad news for your health.

Consider for a moment that just one super-sized soft drink can contain as many as 800 calories. That's about a third of the daily caloric requirement for a large man. One super-sized meal can contain as many as 2,000 calories! On top of that, as a society, we snack almost constantly and wash those snacks down with sugary sodas and fruit drinks. According to the USDA, sugar and sweetener consumption has climbed from and average of 113 pounds per person in 1966 to nearly 150 pounds per person in 2001. The easy accessibility of food has allowed people to snack throughout the day on foods that are for the most part nutrient deficient and loaded with calories. And don't be fooled by diet sodas either. Tests have shown that they can actually lead to weight gain because they don't satisfy thirst and actually create hunger. Not to mention, the artificial sweeteners contained within them are very unhealthy as well.

The flip side of our addiction to unhealthy food is our sedentary lifestyle. For instance, most Americans sit in their cars for transportation to and from a job where they sit for eight hours. Then at lunch, they sit for another hour, during which they eat fast or processed food. After arriving back home they eat even more processed food (and don't forget the junk food snacks after lunch) and then sit in front of a television set or computer until they go to bed, only to rise up the next morning and repeat the insanity.

Our kids are affected as well. In the past, kids would go outside and play after lunch or dinner. They'd climb trees, play tag, and jump rope. Now, they play computer games or watch TV.

This sedentary lifestyle is not only a caloric nightmare, but it also contributes to lower metabolism, which promotes weight gain. Now, to be fair, I understand that a percentage of people do have more active lifestyles or manual jobs. But compared to people of the past, ours is an extremely sedentary culture with poor eating habits.

Consider life as recently as the turn of the century. With no gas-powered vehicles or electricity, nearly everything people did during the day involved some form of exercise. In addition, nearly all the foods eaten were natural. Fast food and junk food simply didn't exist. If you needed to go somewhere, you most likely walked or rode a horse, which was exercise in itself. During the early 1900s, Americans who lived in both small towns and cities alike walked an average of two miles to and from work or school every day, in addition to whatever exercise they did on the job. Life in general included so much more physical labor. Take cleaning house, for example: There were no vacuum cleaners, so women swept their entire houses with a broom and carried the heavy rugs outside to beat the dust out of them. Housework back then was a full body workout!

No doubt, developments in modern medicine have helped lengthen our life spans considerably. Health care has never been more advanced than it is today. We've all but eradicated diseases such as polio and smallpox. Modern medicine has, for the most part, eliminated the possibility of outbreaks of major plagues like those that killed millions upon millions throughout history.

On the other hand, however, our technological advancements have created a modern lifestyle that is killing us. All the conveniences and accessibility have made us fat and unhealthy. Bottom line, Americans are eating more, eating wrong, and exercising less—a deadly combination.

In a July 16, 2004 article, *The Washington Times* reported that "obesity is a critical public health problem in our country that causes millions of Americans to suffer unnecessary health problems and to die prematurely." On April 20, 2005, The *San Francisco Chronicle* reported that "poor diet and lack of exercise still rank as the nation's No. 2 preventable killer behind smoking cigarettes." According to Dr. Jennifer Zebrack, Assistant Professor of Medicine at the Medical College of Wisconsin, "Obesity is the most common nutritional disorder in the developed world."

> **PRACTICAL TIP #2**
> Rethink portion size. When eating out, order half orders or split meals with friends. At home, invest in storage tubs and save half your dinner for lunch the next day.

In addition to not looking or feeling your best, being overweight or obese contributes to the following:

- High blood pressure and high blood cholesterol

- Coronary heart disease, stroke, congestive heart failure

- Type 2 diabetes

- Osteoarthritis

- Gallstones

- Slow metabolism: People who are overweight have a hard time burning off food. As a result fat is stored.

- Build up of toxins in the body

- Low back problems

- Heartburn

- Gout

- Obstructive sleep apnea and other respiratory problems

- Some types of cancer, including breast, prostate, and colon

- Complications of pregnancy

- Poor female reproductive health such as menstrual irregularities and infertility

- Bladder control problems

- Psychological disorders including depression, eating disorders, distorted body image, and low self-esteem

Looking at all of these implications of obesity, we can readily see the staggering problem facing America. We are eating ourselves to death and raising kids who are following in our footsteps! But you don't have to follow the deadly pattern. You have the power to change. You can lose weight, get healthy, and start looking and feeling better today. Even if you feel you have a genetic disposition towards heaviness, you can still lose weight and be healthy.

You may be saying something like, "My whole family is overweight. My mother was overweight. All my aunts are overweight. It's obviously genetic. There is nothing I can do about it." Wrong, wrong, wrong. Science has proven that only 25% of your metabolism is determined by your genes. The other 75% is totally in your control.[1] The vast majority of the time, what we assume is family genetics is actually family behavior and eating patterns that have been handed down from generation to generation.

Dr. Frank Vinicor, director of the Centers for Disease Control and Prevention, said concerning America's problem with weight, "These national increases have more to do with lifestyle than genetic makeup. It isn't our genes that have suddenly changed. What has changed is our society."

The good news is, by developing healthy eating habits and getting regular exercise, you can actually overcome your genes. Physician Lesley Campbell says, "Being active can trump genetics when it comes to staying lean." Regardless of your background, you have the power to take control of your physical destiny. You can change your behavior and make a lifestyle change. And that's the key to long term results: changing our lifestyle.

SUCCESS IN THEIR OWN WORDS:

Billie's Story

- Age thirty-nine, married, one child
- Lost fifty pounds

It all started for me when I was buying clothes for a vacation to Mexico. Trying on all those clothes really got me depressed. I couldn't believe how awful my body looked. When I got home, I dumped emotionally on my husband. To my surprise he didn't belittle me, but encouraged me instead. He asked me, "If you are so miserable with your body, why don't you do something about it? People do it all the time."

Then, on my next trip to the store, I happened across a book full of stories of people who had lost weight and dramatically reshaped their bodies.

Standing right there in the book aisle, tears

*came to my eyes as I flipped through the pages
looking at example after example of people who
had transformed their lives. It was then I decided
to do something about my own life. That was over
five years, fifty pounds, and four dress sizes ago,
and I feel great! It's hard to describe the high you
experience when you see the pounds start to
come off.*

Billie's Eating Habits:

- I try not to have my "weakest" foods in the house.

- I realized that if I wanted to lose weight and keep it from creeping back on, I would have to change the way I ate forever.

- I drink a lot of water to flush my system and keep my muscles hydrated.

- I treat myself at least once a week to something I like to eat.

- I keep a food journal tracking everything I eat throughout the day. This helps me pinpoint my weak areas.

- A typical breakfast is something like oatmeal, egg whites, and a bagel with a touch of low fat cream cheese.

- For a typical lunch, I'll eat grilled or baked chicken, dark green vegetables, and brown rice.

- A typical dinner is lean steak, chicken, or fish with spinach or broccoli and a green leaf salad with fat-free dressing.

- For snacks or mini meals, I fix a protein shake or eat a variety of fruit. I keep a fruit bowl full at home and on my desk at work. I'm always nibbling on fruit.

Billie's Exercise Habits:

- I do fifty minutes of an intense walk/run combination four times a week.

- A lot of times I do aerobics with music. It mixes things up a bit and still gets my heart rate up.

- I try to do strength/resistance exercises for upper and lower body two or three days a week—never less than one day a week. I have found just doing strength training one day a week consistently can have profound results.

PERSONAL REFLECTION:

What do you think most needs to change about your approach to diet and exercise? Do you think it will be hard to begin to do things differently than your family and friends?

YOUR TO DO LIST:

Today, get rid of all the soda in your house. Then go take another walk.

FOR FURTHER STUDY:

Thin Within: A Grace-Oriented Approach to Lasting Weight Loss
—by Judy Wardell Halliday and
Arthur W. Halliday with Heidi Bylsma

How Healthy or Unhealthy Are You—Really?

Weight reduction is not easy, but it doesn't have to be a painful or even a hungry experience. It is a long-term project, and it will be successful only on that basis. Short-term gains and losses are relatively unimportant.

—JAMES M. FERGUSON, M.D.

POWER STATEMENT:

Losing weight in a healthy way is not about pounds lost or conforming to extreme standards of beauty, but about having a healthy body.

When determining your particular health status and whether or not you need to lose weight, the first thing you need to do is throw out those Hollywood supermodel images you might be carrying around. More often than not, you are seeing a distortion of reality. The international supermodel Cindy Crawford once said, "Even I don't wake up looking like Cindy Crawford." Now, having said that, it is quite possible for you to look fit and trim, have a nice figure, and experience optimal health. Just get out of your head trying to look perfect because that will never happen. Everyone has flaws. You can, however look like the person you were created by God to be.

There are two primary ways of determining if you need to lose weight or not. The first is to measure your body mass index, or BMI. When measuring your BMI, use the following formula. Take your body weight in pounds and multiply it by 703. Then divide that number by your height in inches squared (your height in inches times your height in inches). Let's practice on a woman who is five-foot-five and weighs 157 pounds.

157 x 703 = 110371

110371 ÷ 4225 (65 inches times 65 inches) = 26.1

This woman's BMI is 26.1. If your BMI is in the range of 19 to 24.9, you are considered to be at a healthy weight. If your BMI falls between 25 and 29.9, you are considered to be overweight and may incur moderate health risks. If your BMI is above 30, you are considered to be obese. Obesity is associated with increased risk of cancer, heart disease, and other health problems. A BMI of 30 or higher increases the risk of premature death by 50 to 100 percent. If your BMI is over 35 and you have a waist size of over 40 inches (men) or 35 inches (women), you are considered to be at especially high risk for health problems.

Another way to determine how much weight to lose is to consult the following chart based on height and weight.

PRACTICAL TIP #3

Determine how much weight you really need to lose by calculating your body mass index or consulting an ideal weight chart. This will give you a realistic, tangible goal.

Once you have determined your individual weight status, write down your present weight and BMI on a calendar or in your planner or journal. Be sure to date the entry. Next, write down your ideal weight and ideal BMI beside it and then circle it. This is your goal which the rest of this book is going to help you attain. At this point we are not interested in setting a time frame to lose the weight, because our goal is lifestyle change in order to achieve optimal health rather than quick weight loss. One of the benefits of optimal health is you will naturally

Ideal Weight Chart Men's Healthy Weight Range			
Height	Ideal Weight	Low	High
5	106	95	117
5'1"	112	101	123
5'2"	118	106	130
5'3"	124	112	136
5'4"	130	117	143
5'5"	136	122	150
5'6"	142	128	156
5'7"	148	133	163
5'8"	154	139	169
5'9"	160	144	176
5'10"	166	149	183
5'11"	172	155	189
6	178	160	196
6'1"	184	166	202
6'2"	190	171	209
6'3"	196	176	216
6'4"	202	182	222
6'5"	208	187	229
6'6"	214	193	235

Ideal Weight Chart Women's Healthy Weight Range			
Height	Ideal Weight	Low	High
4'7	75	68	83
4'8	80	72	88
4'9	85	77	94
4'10	90	81	99
4'11	95	86	105
5	100	90	110
5'1"	105	95	116
5'2"	110	99	121
5'3"	115	104	127
5'4"	120	108	132
5'5"	125	113	138
5'6"	130	117	143
5'7"	135	122	149
5'8"	140	126	154
5'9"	145	131	160
5'10"	150	135	165
5'11"	155	140	171
6	160	144	176

(**Important Note:** Both the BMI and ideal weight chart will not be accurate for those individuals with high muscle mass. Muscular people will have a higher BMI and a heavier weight although still fit.)

gravitate towards your ideal weight. You should strive for weight loss as a result of healthy habits.

Remember, choose to lose, but don't diet. Dieting is the counterfeit to real healthy living. As I've previously stated in Chapter 1, in order to achieve this goal of optimal health, of looking and feeling better, it will require changing our thinking about food and exercise and then developing new habits to replace the old ones. The rest of this book is divided into two parts. Part I deals with the nutritional aspect of weight loss and Part II deals with the exercise aspect. Now, let's go for it!

SUCCESS IN THEIR OWN WORDS:

Alice's Story

- Age thirty-seven, divorced, three children
- Lost eighty-five pounds and went from a size twenty-two to a size eight

I became unhappy with my weight after the birth of my third baby. It was important to me that I be able to do activities with my children. To lose my weight, I changed my eating habits and joined a health club where the owner put me on a workout routine. Probably the most difficult thing for me to do was go to the club as fat as I was. It was very embarrassing and humbling. But the people there were very supportive, and I was determined. After about two months, I started seeing small results. I built on each little success that I had. When I started out I weighed over 250 pounds. Now, I weigh 165! That was over five years ago and I have maintained that weight.

Alice's Eating Habits:

- I keep a diet journal of what I am eating so I can keep track of my calories.

- I drink lots of water.

- I try to stay positive and focused and refuse to listen to the naysayers. Try to find friends who will encourage and support you

Alice's Exercise Habits:

- I planned my exercise regimen into my daily schedule.

- I do machines and free weights, lower and upper body.

- I began by walking, then began jogging three miles four days a week.

- I often take Pilates classes at the club.

PERSONAL REFLECTION:

How much weight do you want to lose? How much do you think you should lose? When you think about losing weight, do you think mostly in terms of looking a certain way, or in terms of being healthy?

YOUR TO DO LIST:

Calculate your BMI and check where you stand on the ideal weight chart. How much weight do you need to lose?

FOR FURTHER STUDY:

Do I Look Fat in This? Life Doesn't Begin Five Pounds from Now
—by Jessica Weiner

Weight Watchers Family Power: Five Simple Rules for a Healthy-Weight Home
—by Karen Miller-Kovach

PART I

CHANGING OUR THINKING ABOUT NUTRITION

CHAPTER 4

The Incredible Impact of Small, Consistent Choices

The key to weight loss and healthy living is in the little choices you make everyday. Consistent, small choices really add up over the long haul.

—LYDIA FELLNER, RN

POWER STATEMENT:

When we're trying to lose weight, we can't overestimate the power of small choices if we're committed and persistent in developing new habits.

I once heard a comedian say, "If you eat fat and greasy food, you will become a fat and greasy dude." That may be a tough statement to hear, but it's dead-on true. You really are what you eat, and just like a computer or an automobile, the human body performs based on what we put into it. If we put damaging things into our bodies, the body will respond accordingly. However, if we put into our body good things, it will respond positively and begin to cleanse and heal itself.

For a moment, try and think how you would treat your automobile if you were allowed only one per lifetime. If that one car had to last your whole life, I'm quite certain you would treat it with extra, ongoing care—keeping it clean, waxing it, changing the oil and the filters, and giving it tune-ups regularly. You would only put in the best gas and the best oil. Well, each of us only gets one body that has to last us our entire lifetime. Yet most of us treat our vehicles with greater care and respect than we do our own bodies.

Unlike the human body, when a vehicle is in need of refurbishing, it can be done fairly quickly—an entire motor can be rebuilt in a week. But that's not so with the human body. Making positive, lasting changes to the human body takes time. It's a process. In fact, changing too fast can actually have harmful and adverse effects on our systems.

In other words, there are no quick ways to long-term gains (or losses). Usually when someone pursues rapid weight loss, at some point they will go off the diet and eventually end up gaining the weight back, plus some. After years of yo-yo dieting, a person can wind up in worse condition, weighing much more than when they started dieting in the first place. We pursue all kinds of things in an attempt to achieve rapid weight loss: fad diets or extremely low-calorie diets, diet pills, fat burning supplements, laxatives, or even gimmicky fitness devices or programs that promise incredible results in little time with little effort. Like the old saying goes, if it sounds too good to be true, it probably is.

The road to long-term weight loss and optimum health is paved with small day-to-day changes that add up over time. Small, consistent changes equal lasting results. Take the area of calorie consumption, for example. Consuming just 250 fewer calories per day can translate into a one-pound weight loss in a week. Most of us consume unnecessary calories without even thinking about it. But simply being aware and making minor adjustments can make major differences. Trimming 250 calories from your daily diet can be as simple as skipping the French fries at lunch or eating only a couple bites of the piece of pie instead of the whole slice. If you order a Junior Whopper instead of the Whopper at Burger King, that will save you about 350 calories. Drinking skim milk instead of whole milk cuts about 100 calories from an eight-ounce glass. Switching from regular salad dressing to low fat can save around 120 calories per tablespoon.

See how small adjustments can really add up over the long haul? Rapid, shortcut gimmicks equal poor health and disappointment. By staying consistent with the small changes, gradually implementing more changes over time, at some point a residual effect begins to take place. It's a point when everything you are doing eventually mushrooms. Remember, what you do in the present has a direct impact on how you will live tomorrow. It's called preventative medicine.

PRACTICAL TIP #4

Find one area where you can cut calories. Cut out soda, eat veggies or crackers at lunch instead of potato chips, or stop frying food.

If you want to lose weight, feel and look better, and experience optimum health over the long haul, there are small—but critical—choices to be made each and every day, leading to the development of improved habits. Now, you'll get no argument from me that changing any habit, particularly eating, is a difficult challenge. And it's even more challenging if you're expecting overnight results. When progress seems to be going too slow and you're tempted to give up, you must realize that what took many years to develop can't be undone in a week or a month. The eating habits you are attempting to change have taken a lifetime to become ingrained into your makeup. Trying to change them too quickly almost always ends in failure.

When attempting long-term change in eating, it is important to focus on developing positive habits rather than trying to defeat the embedded negative ones. Don't focus on stopping the negatives, but on replacing them with positive ones. Most of the time it's much easier to implement new habits than to suddenly drop the old ones. As a new habit becomes a part of your daily life, the intensity of the old one naturally lessens and eventually disappears.

Now it's time to see what kind of positive habits we need to develop to experience weight loss and optimal health.

SUCCESS IN THEIR OWN WORDS:

Sarah's Story

- Age thirty-four, married with two children, ages twelve and eight
- Lost thirty-two pounds and went from a size ten to a size two

When I viewed the pictures from our ten-year family reunion, I was in shock. I knew I had put on weight, but seeing the pictures opened my eyes to how overweight I really was. I became so depressed because I didn't want to be a fat wife and mother. After about a week, something clicked inside of me. It's like I just knew something had to change and I had to start right then or I would continue to gain more weight.

I read everything I good get my hands on about weight loss and came to the understanding that I had to start exercising and completely alter the way I was eating. The books really confirmed something that I already knew internally. Because of our fast-paced lifestyle with the kids, we ate lots of fast food and pizza. One of my first changes was to cut out the junk food and make healthier food choices for the whole family.

It did not take me long to get addicted to exercise, but the nutritional aspect was much harder. When I didn't see results as quickly as I wanted, or would have a setback, I would get discouraged and want to give up. But I literally forced myself to keep going. I told myself: stick with *it for at least six months before you quit the program.*

Well, after those six months I couldn't believe how much better I felt and much better my clothes fit me. Then, a couple months after that, the weight really began to come off. It took me over a year to lose to my present weight and I have kept it off for three years now. My habits have completely changed. I work out at least four days a week and eat healthy on a consistent basis.

The old me is gone—I'm a totally new person, more contented and more confident, attempting things that I never would have considered before. My husband and children are thrilled with the new me, but I think I'm happier than any of them!

Sarah's Eating Habits:

- I recognized my weaknesses with food and took those items out of my house. If the ice cream isn't there, I can't eat it!

- I snack before I get hungry. I try to eat a small snack every couple of hours throughout the day, which helps curbs my appetite so I eat smaller meals. If I let myself get really hungry, it's harder for me to keep from eating junk food.

- I do a little research before I eat out. Most restaurants now have their nutrition information posted online, so I check it out beforehand. I am much less likely to eat something if I know how fattening it really is.

- I give myself one "free" day a week for eating. If you know you can eat whatever you want on that day, it makes it easier to stick with your plan the rest of the week. Eat what you want, but don't overeat.

- I've learned to eat smaller portions. It's never a good idea to overeat, even with healthy foods.

Sarah's Exercise Habits:

- I do strength training twice a week for about thirty minutes and run three times a week for forty-five minutes.

PERSONAL REFLECTION:

What small changes can you make in your day-to-day life to optimize your health? What choices have you been putting off?

YOUR TO DO LIST:

Choose one small change you can make to your dieting habits—set a goal to eat five fruits and vegetables every day or drink eight glasses of water.

FOR FURTHER STUDY:

Look Great, Feel Great: Twelve Keys to Enjoying a Healthy Life Now
—by Joyce Meyer

Good Food Has the Power

The only way to change your body is to eat.
You can never get lean, shrink, or be the size you
want to be if you don't eat. Diets don't work.
I beg you—stop dieting forever.
Food does not make you fat. Fat makes you fat.

—SUSAN POWTER

POWER STATEMENT:

> In order to lose weight and be at our best, we don't need to turn away from food, but turn to the right kinds of food to help us.

I f you're going to lose weight in a healthy, lasting way, something that must become ingrained in your thinking is that good food has the power. Good food actually balances your system and promotes health, whereas bad food creates unbalance and kills. Just as irrevocable damage is done when a smoker inhales a puff of smoke, when you take in bad food, your body suffers damage. However, in the same way, when you take in good food, your body thrives.

Consuming good food empowers you in a number of ways. Good food increases your energy level while decreasing your chances of developing illnesses such as diabetes, cancer, heart disease, and stroke. Developing good eating habits in combination with proper exercise helps your appearance as well, and not only your shape, but also your hair, skin, fingernails, and other features. Those who eat well tend to have a more youthful look and age better than poor eaters.

And besides all that, eating healthy food facilitates weight loss because when you eat the right food, your calorie intake naturally goes down or balances to the proper level. You can eat more and feel full with fewer calories. And in order to lose weight, it's important to reduce calories—but not by dieting. That may sound like a contradictory statement, but it's not. When eating right, you can eat more for less. Take fresh cherries or grapes, for example. These guys can really satisfy a craving for sweets. If you grab a candy bar in response to a sweet tooth attack, you can knock down 300 calories in a few seconds. You'd have to eat a pile of cherries or grapes to blow through that many calories at once. Plus, because you'll eat them more slowly than you would a candy bar, you'll feel fuller when finished. Research has shown that foods eaten quickly tend to aid weight gain because the body doesn't have the time it needs to let the feeling of fullness take over. (Plus, both cherries and grapes have other benefits, too. A cup of cherries provides almost 25 percent of the Recommended Dietary Allowance of Vitamin A. Cherries and grapes are also good for the heart. Good food is good all around!)

PRACTICAL TIP #5

When craving sweets, snack on fresh or frozen fruit.

Most processed and fast foods are thick with calories because they contain excessive amounts of fat. A unit of fat contains nine calories, while a unit of carbohydrates and proteins contain only four. Foods that are high in nutrition value are usually lower in fat and sugar, so they're lower in calories. So by choosing the correct foods, it is possible to increase your consumption and lose weight at the same time. The secret is to modify your eating habits so that you get the most value for each calorie—to get more nutritional bang for your buck, so to speak. Reduce your fat and sugar intake and eat more fruits and vegetables, and you automatically reduce your calorie consumption.

Put simply, you can eat more, fill up, feel satisfied, and still lose weight if you eat the right foods. In time, you will transform an overweight, unhealthy body into one that is stronger, leaner, and more attractive.

The Dangers of Dieting

When a person diets instead of dealing with the root problems of weight gain, they are really only treating the symptoms. Dieting becomes a battle of willpower, and when battling willpower, hunger usually wins out, leaving the dieter feeling guilty or weak. Self-esteem plummets, depression sets in, and many times binging takes place. But the whole battle was based on a lie, on false information. The truth is, when we are hungry, we should eat until we are full. Eating is natural and healthy. Starving yourself is not.

What happens to the human body when you deprive yourself of food for a period of time is that your body begins to yearn for high-calorie foods. Please understand that when this happens you shouldn't feel guilty, weak, or like you have no willpower. Your body is doing what it is supposed to do, reacting to starvation. It's attempting to function properly but can't find any fuel. Your body is pleading with you to give it some gas so it can keep going! A person's willpower may last for a few weeks or months, but eventually they give in to binge eating. In this case, binging is not an eating disorder; it's the body's attempt to stay alive.

When you eat good food, the calories are lower, but your body does not go into starvation mode, so you don't binge. Eventually, your body adapts to good food and starts to crave healthy things instead of unhealthy things.

If you persist with an excessively low-calorie diet, your body will say, "If you are not going to give me food, I'll just find it elsewhere." And, that's exactly what it does. Because your body is not getting enough fuel to function on, it starts feeding on lean muscle mass, which is not a good for you. It's not good because when you lose weight from lean muscle mass, and gain it back, like most on diets eventually do, the lost muscle comes back as fat, which causes more weight gain and more health problems. You need muscles to burn calories. A single pound of resting muscle burns fifty calories per day, compared to a pound of fat which burns a whopping three calories! We will see in Part II more of why muscle mass plays an important role in weight loss and optimal health.

In addition to feeding on muscle mass, excessive dieting slows down the metabolic rate, which further inhibits body's ability to burn fat and calories. Diets don't work. They zap your energy and leave you tired, hungry, and often heavier.

It must become entrenched in our minds that eating good food does not make people fat. Food is energy for life. It's essential for good health. In order to get fit, you have to eat. True, you must eat the right foods, but reaching your ideal weight and health requires that you eat. There's no way around it. This is why we must develop new positive habits instead of merely battling to say no to

PRACTICAL TIP #6

Erase the word "diet" from your vocabulary, as long as "dieting" means temporarily depriving yourself of certain foods. Instead, build healthy foods into your daily eating habits, and allow yourself treats every now and then.

negative ones. Remember, we are changing our thinking, switching to a new paradigm, and sometimes that is more difficult than we initially thought. As we discussed in the previous chapter, success comes in developing the small, consistent daily habits. Developing habits of eating good food has the power to bring long term weight loss and alter our lives. Consider Jim's story. His is a compelling testimony to the transforming power of good food.

Jim is an amazing character. At seventy-four years old, he has so much energy that you can barely keep up with him. He never lets up. His life is filled with vision and zest. He owns a beautiful 300-acre farm with over 200 head of beef cattle. Owning a business in the city, it was his lifelong dream to retire on the farm, and after thirty years of hard work, he finally got his wish.

Now, tending a 300-acre cattle ranch is not for the weak in body. It's a full time and highly physical job for a young man, must less a seventy-four-year-old. But don't tell that to Jim. He'll just ignore you and get on with his work. He shows no signs of slowing down. Jim said, "I feel so youthful that sometimes it surprises me when I look in the mirror and realize that I'm as old as I am." Then he laughed, "That's why I don't look in the mirror too much."

To give you an idea of the shape Jim is in, when I was with him visiting, he was unloading fifty- and hundred-pound sacks of feed out of his truck. He was tossing them up on his back and then stacking them. Not one or two sacks, but twenty or thirty. He'd just finished building a 4000-square-foot barn on the property, doing most of the construction himself. Yes, I mean climbing on the up rafters and laying tin roofing, hammering, heavy lifting, digging trenches, and pouring concrete. Friends and relatives helped, but Jim outworked them all. The guy is amazing!

Jim's body is mean and lean, and just a few days before I wrote this chapter, his doctor informed him that his heart, kidneys, prostate, and blood pressure were all perfect. So what is Jim's secret? You'd be surprised. Is it genetics? No. His secret is good food and a lot of exercise. And here's why I make that claim—

You see, Jim has not always been the picture of good health. In fact, on a couple of occasions, he almost died. About twenty

> ## PRACTICAL TIP #7
> Get started. You don't have to rearrange your entire life tomorrow— start with developing one healthy eating habit, then another, then another. The important thing is that you do something.

years ago, Jim found out that he had adult-onset diabetes. The day his blood sugar shot up to almost 700, he went into a semi-coma. At the time, he was overweight and had engaged in a lifetime of poor eating habits. The doctor told him to either change his eating habits or die. It was that simple. Jim's condition did not require insulin, but it did require a very strict no sugar, low-fat eating regimen. With the help of his wife, Nell, Jim cut his fat intake and went cold turkey off sugars. Nell and Jim began educating themselves about the power of eating right. Giving up all that sugar and fat sounds like such a hard life. But don't you dare feel sorry for Jim. He wouldn't go back to his old way of life for anything.

Eventually, his body shed over thirty excess pounds, his blood sugar stabilized, and his energy level sky rocketed. Jim started feeling really outstanding, not only physically but mentally as well—like he could conquer the world. And Jim has conquered his world.

His regimen of eating right was no temporary thing. It was a lifelong program. It had to be. If he were to eat the wrong foods his blood sugar would go back up and his health would plummet. As hard as it is to believe, for over twenty years, Jim has eaten almost zero processed sugar. Sure, the adjustment was difficult at first, but eventually he arrived at the point where he actually turns his nose up at the taste of sugar. It's too sweet. His body now craves natural, whole foods.

If changing his way of eating and thinking about food revolutionized Jim's life with diabetes, how much more could it do for you? Don't wait for diabetes, heart disease, or some other illness to hit before you take action. You have the power within yourself to develop the positive habits that will lead to a slimmer, leaner, and healthier you, starting right now.

PERSONAL REFLECTION:

What kind of relationship do you have with healthy food? Did you grow up eating more Cheetos than vegetables? Do you find yourself often suspicious of "health nuts" and the kind of foods they enjoy?

YOUR TO DO LIST:

This week, don't focus on what not to eat—focus on what good foods you should eat. Pick five healthy foods you enjoy and work them into your diet each day this week.

FOR FURTHER STUDY:

Body by God: The Owner's Manual for Maximized Living
—by Ben Lerner

So What Do I Eat to Lose Weight and Be Healthy?

Eating to lose body fat—it sounds too good to be true! Yet, not only is it true, it is the only way to successfully lose body-fat and keep it off.

—CLIFF SHEATS

POWER STATEMENT:

By getting the right amount of the right foods into our daily diets, we're well on our way to a trim, healthy body.

We know it matters how we eat. We know good food is our ally in the fight for a healthy body. But what does a healthy diet look like? Let's look at some principles of eating for weight loss.

Calories Do Count

Eating the correct amount of calories is important to optimal health, and cutting calories is usually necessary to weight loss. Regardless of who you are, if you take in more calories than you burn, you will gain weight. If you burn more calories than you take in, you will lose weight. However, and this is important, you never want to go below your base calorie requirements.

To find out the total number of calories your body needs per day, you can use the following formula to calculate your approximate RMR (Resting Metabolic Rate). Your RMR is the base number of calories your body needs to function properly. Again, let's use a thirty-year-old woman who is five-foot-five in height and weighs 157 pounds as an example.

Formula:

655 + (4.4 times weight in pounds) + (4.7 times height in inches) − (4.7 times age) = 1510.3

Next, to establish actual daily caloric needs, factor in your activity level by multiplying the RMR (1510.3) by a figure from one of the categories below:

- 0.9 if you are inactive and have crash dieted frequently over the two years

- 1.2 if you are inactive

- 1.3 if you are moderately active (three days per week or equivalent)

- 1.7 if you are very active

- 1.9 if extremely active

This formula should be considered for normal daily body function, not weight loss. To lose weight, subtract 300-500 calories per day from your total energy needs.

We've already seen that eating too little, skipping meals, and excessively cutting calories can send the body into starvation mode. To keep your metabolism high and your hunger in check, eat regular meals and consume at least your base RMR calories. Remember, the key to long-term weight loss is the combination of eating right and exercise that burns excess calories.

PRACTICAL TIP #8

Do the math. Determine how many calories you need to eat in order to maintain your weight, and how many you need to eat in order to lose weight.

What and How to Eat

Good nutrition absolutely does not mean a sacrifice in flavor. Here are some ideas on building healthy foods into your diet.

- Vary the vegetables. Eat more dark green vegetables such as spinach, broccoli, and other dark leafy greens; orange vegetables, such as carrots, sweet potatoes, pumpkin, and winter squash; and beans and peas, such as pinto beans, kidney beans, black beans, garbanzo beans, split peas, and lentils. Just look around your local zoo and you'll see plenty of animals that have grown to good size on diets exclusively herbivorous: horses, bison, elephants, cattle, gorillas, giraffes, and other imposing creatures. Man has the option of going either way—meat or no meat. As with just about everything else in life, extremes in diet should be avoided. And remember that your dietary scales should weigh heavily on the vegetable and fruit side.

- Get friendly with fruits. Eat a variety of fruits, whether fresh, frozen, canned, or dried. Eating whole fruit is better than fruit juice. A good rule of thumb is two cups of fruit each day. For example: one banana, one large orange, and half a cup of peaches.

- Make half your grains whole. Eat at least three ounces of whole-grain cereals, breads, crackers, rice, or pasta every day. One ounce is about one slice of bread, one cup of breakfast cereal, or half a cup of cooked rice or pasta. Look to see that grains such as wheat, rice, oats, or corn are referred to as "whole" in the list of ingredients.

• Go lean with protein. Choose lean meats and poultry. Bake it, broil it, or grill it. Vary your protein choices with more fish, beans, peas, nuts, and seeds. You don't have to include animal-based foods (meat, poultry, fish, and dairy) to have a healthy diet. But, on the other hand, eating these foods is not incompatible with health as long as you don't overdo it.

PRACTICAL TIP #9

Lose the frying pan. Bake or broil, steam or stir fry your meats and vegetables instead of frying.

• Limit saturated fats. Get less than 20 to 30 percent of calories from fats. Most fats should come from sources of polyunsaturated and monounsaturated fatty acids, such as fish, nuts, and vegetable oils. When selecting and preparing meat, poultry, dry beans, and milk or milk products, make choices that are lean, low-fat, or fat-free.

• Get your calcium-rich foods. Get three cups of low-fat or fat-free milk—or an equivalent amount of low-fat yogurt or low-fat cheese— every day. If you don't or can't consume milk, choose lactose-free milk products or calcium-fortified foods and drinks.

- Limit salt. Get less than one teaspoon of salt each day. Try vegetable salt and salt substitutes. They work great!

- Reduce your intake of refined sugar. Most foods high in refined sugar are high in calories but devoid of nutritional value. It is better to leave out sugar all together or limit it to a nominal amount if you desire to effectively control your weight and maximize your energy.

PRACTICAL TIP #10

Cut sugar cravings by making sure your breakfast includes some protein, and balancing protein, carbohydrates, and fats in each meal. With a few well-placed snacks and plenty of water, you'll probably find that your sweet tooth is much more easily satisfied.

- Limit partially hydrogenated fats to an absolute minimum. This is the process by which liquid vegetable oils are hardened into semi-solid fats for use in processed food and fast-food frying. These oils have adverse effects and offer no counter-balancing nutritional benefits.

- Broil, bake, roast, stir fry, or steam instead of deep-fat frying. When you skip the deep-fried foods, you not only make a significant dent in your fat intake, but you also avoid potentially cancerous elements.

Eating out and Staying Fit— You Can Do It

The author Joyce Meyer once said, "Quality decisions must be made if we are to take charge of our bodies. I got rid of my bad food habits by making the commitment that every piece of food I put in my mouth would be a conscious decision." According to her, mindful eating is "simply being present—really present—whenever you choose to put food or drink in your mouth." Well, this concept is especially true when we eat out. It is possible to have success eating out, but only if we are mindful eaters. By being mindful of our surroundings, what we will find is that we really do have several options available. The following are some painless ways to find nutritional success at restaurants:

- Just say no to super sizing. The size you ordered is already too big. Stop super sizing and you'll save money.

- Share a meal. You save calories and money.

- Stop ordering drinks with your meals and drink water.

- Watch portion sizes and ask for a to-go box at the start of the meal. When your meal is served, immediately measure off some to take home. Most restaurants in the United States serve way too much.

- Get a copy of the restaurant's nutritional guide and see how many calories you are really eating. This can often be found online.

- Just say no to bread and rolls. Why fill up on ordinary bread when you're paying good money for a meal? Just ask the server to take it away.

- Plan ahead. Have an idea of what you want to eat before arriving at the restaurant and order the healthiest and leanest entrees. When possible, avoid looking at the menu so as not to be tempted with other food choices.

- Restrict alcohol consumption. Alcohol spoils healthy eating by increasing the appetite and adding needless calories.

PRACTICAL TIP #11

When eating out, look for healthy options. Eat half of what the restaurant serves you, and substitute vegetables or fruit for fries or coleslaw.

- Share dessert. If you have a sweet tooth and really want dessert, share it with a friend.

- No restaurants are banned. These days, well-informed food choices can be made at just about every restaurant or fast-food establishment.

- Order broiled, baked, or grilled instead of fried.

- Order off the kids' menu. Get the same food in smaller quantity, which means fewer calories.

- Order a three portion meal. Begin with a light non-cream based soup; then order a salad with dressing on the side; followed by a leaner cut of meat and eat a smaller portion.

A Word about Supplements

I am a firm believer in vitamin and nutritional supplements. However, it is important to understand that the word "supplement" means just that: a supplement, not a replacement. The American Dietetic Association said, "The best nutritional strategy for promoting optimal health and reducing risk of chronic disease is to obtain adequate nutrients from a wide variety of foods." They recommend vitamin supplements as a second alternative.[1]

> **PRACTICAL TIP #12**
>
> Snack smart. As you decrease your portion sizes, you won't even notice that you're eating half as much at mealtime if you eat a few smart snacks throughout the day.

If you find yourself missing some of the important nutrients that the body needs, it would be better to take a supplement than to miss out on the benefits of that nutrient altogether. When you take supplements, make sure you take ones that absorb into to your system easily. Don't cut costs on vitamins, because you usually get what you pay for. My experience has been that powders and liquids absorb more effectively than pills.

PRACTICAL TIP #13

Plan ahead. When you do your grocery shopping, stock up on plenty of healthy staples and steer clear of the junk food aisle.

As I said above, eating healthy does not mean eating blah. If you've always thought of healthy food as bland, boring cardboard, think again. As you learn new ways to cook and eat, you'll find yourself loving food more than you ever have before.

14 Surefire Tips for Weight Loss and Nutritional Success

- Keep a journal to record your eating and physical activity. Write down your goals, progress, and disappointments. Reviewing the journal will help you measure progress and determine where you might need to change.

- Remember, it's growth, not perfection, that really matters. Momentary slips in healthy eating, exercise, and your attitude aren't failures but opportunities to learn and grow.

- Be a mindful eater. Consider everything that you put in your mouth. You'll find a sample journal starting on page 165. When you grab that candy bar or your hand is in a bag of potato chips, ask yourself why. Mindless eating often occurs while doing something else like watching television, reading, socializing, or cooking. Be alert for emotions or stress that triggers overeating.

- Everything you eat does not have to be bursting with good nutrition. You can enjoy most foods, as long as you follow the principles of balance, variety, and moderation.

- Adjust the amount of food you eat according to the time of day. Eat your bigger meals early and smaller ones later. Try not to eat major meals after 6:00 P.M.

- Know your daily caloric needs for maintaining your ideal weight. Then you can adjust accordingly for weight gain or weight loss.

- View each meal as an opportunity to honor your body and life.

- Value your hunger. Physical hunger is the signal to eat. Eat only until you are comfortably full. Learn to ascertain between legitimate hunger and impulses to eat, which begin with the sight, smell, or thought of food.

- Be aware of what you drink! It's amazing how many extra calories are in sodas, juices, and other drinks. Cutting out soda completely can save you 360 or more calories each day. Avoid diet soda, too. The artificial sweeteners actually make you hungry.

- Drink a complete glass of water before each meal, which will curb your hunger and cause you to eat less.

- Eat slowly so your brain can get the message that your stomach is full. Here's a little trick that helps: It is impossible to eat fast if you set your utensil down after each bite.

- Never, ever skip a meal, especially breakfast.

- Eat smaller portions and always leave a little bit on the plate. At home, always serve food on smaller salad plates and you will get in the habit of eating less. Go ahead and eat desserts, but only take a couple bites instead of the whole piece of pie.

- Clean up your environment. What you don't have around, you won't eat.

PERSONAL REFLECTION:

Do you feel optimistic about building healthy eating habits? How hard or easy do you think it will be to change the way you eat?

✓ YOUR TO DO LIST:

Do the math: Figure out how many calories you need to eat each day to lose weight. A warning: Sometimes calorie-counting can become a bit obsessive and foster feelings of guilt, which will not bring true weight-loss success.

FOR FURTHER STUDY:

The EatingWell Healthy in a Hurry Cookbook:
150 Delicious Recipes for Simple, Everyday Suppers in
45 Minutes or Less
        —by Jim Romanoff and the editors of EatingWell

CHAPTER 7

Water: It Helps with Just About Everything

*Pure water comes closer
to being a genuine health potion
than any other substance on our planet.*

—TED BROER

POWER STATEMENT:

Water is a crucial element
in our quest for healthy bodies.

It's really quite simple. If you want to lose weight and be healthier, drink lots and lots of water. I know, I know—you've heard it a thousand times before. But just because you've heard something time and time again doesn't make it less important. Did you know that drinking enough water each day is one of the most excellent health secrets out there? It's also a major key in weight loss and sustaining weight loss. Yet, because of its simplicity and abundance, a lot of people just pass over its benefits, which are many.

Let's start with the basics. You can live without food for about a month, but only a few days without water. Have you ever wondered why? It's because water accounts for a large percentage of our physical makeup. Nearly two-thirds of our body is water.

- Our blood is 83% water.
- Our muscles are 75% water.
- The brain is 85% water.
- Our lungs are 80% water.

So what do these numbers mean to your overall health? Consider that a decline of only a couple of percentage points in your body's water can prompt short-term memory loss and can cause you to have difficulty focusing and energy loss leading to fatigue. Water is what makes it possible for your body to digest and absorb vital vitamins and nutrients. In addition, it cleanses the liver and kidneys and carries away waste from the body. When dehydrated, the blood becomes thicker, making circulation more difficult, which causes the brain to become lethargic and the body fatigued.

Drinking an abundance of water also reduces the chances of bladder cancer by 50%, colon cancer by 45%, and significantly lessens the risk of breast cancer. If that is not enough, water slows down the aging process. It flushes out impurities in your skin, leaving it clear and radiant. Water does so much for us. It helps:

- Improve energy
- Enhance brain performance
- Enhance physical performance
- Remove toxins and waste
- Keep skin unblemished
- Reduce headaches
- Improve digestion, kidney function, and circulation
- Nurture the body's natural healing mechanisms

How Drinking Water Helps with Weight Loss

First, water creates a sense of fullness, which as a result will make you less inclined to overeat. Also, water is a natural appetite suppressant, so developing a good water drinking habit can be a long-term aid in achieving and maintaining a healthy weight. Frequently, thirst is mistaken for hunger, and instead of reaching for a glass of water, many will grab something to eat. However, if you will drink a glass of water before you eat, quite often you will find that you weren't that hungry after all, just thirsty.

Another important thing water does is assist your body in metabolizing stored fat. Simply put, drinking water

> **PRACTICAL TIP #14**
>
> Drink at least eight glasses of water a day, paying special attention to mealtimes.

increases the metabolic rate, which in turn burns more calories. When not getting a proper water supply, the metabolic rate slows, and it's more difficult for you to turn stored fat into energy, or calories. It does not make sense to take all the time and effort to lose weight, only to retard the process by not adequately hydrating your body. Studies have shown that those that battle obesity are usually poor water drinkers. If you are serious about your quest to become leaner and healthier, then you must also become a serious water drinker.

How Much Water Do I Need to Drink?

Simply put, you need to drink at least eight to ten glasses of water a day. Before meals or snacks, you should drink eight ounces of water. It's really not that difficult to drink an adequate amount of water and reap its benefits. Like everything else we've talked about, it's all about developing habits. Many people fill up a bottle or jug each morning and carry it around with them all day. That's the easiest way to get in the habit. In fact, the majority of people I know who have lost weight and kept it off are big time water drinkers.

Tips to Make Water Drinking Easier

- As much as possible, drink water instead of coffee and sodas that contain caffeine. Caffeine is a diuretic, which means it has a slight dehydrating effect. Caffeine literally forces water out of your system. That's why sodas and coffee never quench your thirst and you always want more. You'll also reap a lot of benefits from replacing sugar- and sweetener-laden beverages with water.

- Drink a big glass of water first thing in the morning. When you wake up, your body is naturally thirsty. This first drink will help flush out the toxins that have been accumulating throughout the night. It's easier to drink a lot of water first thing, so take advantage of this thirst to get ahead on your daily water requirements.

- If you're cold, drink warm water instead of coffee. If at all possible, try to wean yourself off of coffee altogether.

- Set a timer to remind yourself to establish a habit of drinking water, and keep a bottle of water with you at all times.

- Spice it up. Add lemon or lime. You can buy flavored water in bottles—but be careful to check for sugar and artificial sweeteners.

PERSONAL REFLECTION:

How are you doing on water drinking? How do you think your health will improve if you make efforts to drink more water?

☑ YOUR TO DO LIST:

Buy a quart-sized water bottle and start carrying it with you throughout the day. Drink half of it on your way to work and the other half before lunch, then refill. Try to finish your second quart before you leave the office for the day.

FOR FURTHER STUDY:

The Water Prescription: For Health, Vitality, and Rejuvenation
        —by Christopher Vasey

PART II

CHANGING OUR THINKING ABOUT EXERCISE

CHAPTER 8

Something You Can't Live Without

*By taking yourself from a sedentary state,
you can, in effect, reduce your biological age
by ten to twenty years.*

—ROY SHEPHAR, M.D., PH.D.

POWER STATEMENT:

A weight-loss program—or any program for optimal health—is incomplete without exercise.

From the very onset of this section, it is critical that we understand fully the connection between exercise and healthy living. You have probably seen more than your share of infomercials and advertisements touting that you can lose weight without exercise and eat anything you want. Well, I hate to burst your bubble, but if it sounds too good to be true, beware. You may lose weight today, but I guarantee you will not be healthy tomorrow. Without exercise, losing weight and keeping it off is virtually impossible. You can eat all the right foods, drink only water, and take a suitcase full of vitamins and supplements, but if you don't exercise, you will never reach optimal health. Likewise, you can exercise for hours, seven days a week, and poor eating habits will nullify it all. To be optimally healthy—and the key word is "optimally"—it takes a combination of the two. We've already discussed the benefits of proper nutrition. In this section, we're going to look at the benefits of exercise on healthy living.

Now, I realize that whenever the word "exercise" is mentioned, all sorts of images come to mind, from complete drudgery to outright boredom, or a life that consists of slogans like "no pain no gain," of gritting your teeth and pushing through. But a lifestyle of physical fitness doesn't have to look like that. The chief reward of keeping physically fit is an enhanced quality of life— looking better, feeling better, and being able to do things you enjoy for longer periods of time. Quality of life is a major concern to most people as they grow older, and exercise is not about merely surviving in life, but about thriving in life for longer.

Just as exercise is an investment that pays immediate rewards and long-term dividends, it has also been confirmed that that the lack of exercise can be detrimental to a person's health. A recent article in the *Journal of the American Medical Association* revealed that those who do not exercise, when contrasted to those who exercise consistently, could expect their risk of dying prematurely to double.

The good news is, you do not have to be a part of those numbers. But positive change takes a determined choice

> ## PRACTICAL TIP #15
>
> Get smart about exercise. Recognize that exercise is a necessary part of fitness, then do some research and experimenting to figure out which exercises you most enjoy. If exercise is fun, you're more likely to stick with it.

followed by repeated action. To improve the quality of our existence, we must break the tendency of lapsing back into the patterns that keep us unhealthy and ineffective in life. One way to rise above this dilemma is to heighten our body awareness and our physical capability. That happens through a lifestyle change involving consistent exercise. I'm not talking about a quick spurt that will burn you out in a few months, but a slow, steady, building, lifelong commitment. The physical benefits of such a lifestyle change are numerous. Here are just a few.

Twenty-One Ways Exercise Helps You Right Now and Later On

- Exercise causes you to burn more calories, during activity and at rest. This helps you achieve a healthy balance between the calories you take in from food and those you expend. The key to weight control is keeping energy intake (food) and energy output (physical activity) in balance. For example, if you consume 100 calories a day more than your body needs, you will gain approximately 10 pounds in a year. You could take that weight off, or keep it off, by doing thirty minutes of moderate exercise daily.

- Exercise actually diminishes the appetite.

- Exercise tones and strengthens muscles of the arms, legs, and abdomen, which improves endurance and appearance.

- Exercise boosts circulation by expanding blood vessels. This greatly diminishes the risks of heart attack and stroke.

- Exercise builds physical and mental stamina and even slows down the aging process by enhancing the transfer of oxygen and other vital nutrients to the body's cells—the brain and lungs included.

- Exercise lowers blood pressure, which is a

major risk factor for heart attacks, aneurysms, glaucoma, and stroke.

- Exercise has proven itself to be a stress reducer. Cardiologist Robert S. Elliot said, "Exercise appears to burn up excess stress chemicals by using them for energy expressed outwardly rather than inwardly where they can do harm."

- Exercise improves the percentage of good to bad cholesterol in the blood. This also decreases the risk of heart attacks due to arterial blockage caused by the buildup of plaque on artery walls.

- Exercise aids in the body's production and distribution of insulin (how the body processes sugar), thus greatly reducing the risk of type II (adult onset) diabetes.

- Exercise aids digestion and hence optimal absorption of vital nutrients.

- Exercise helps with intestinal regularity, therefore lessening the chances of colon cancer.

- Exercise strengthens bones by increasing their ingestion of calcium, dramatically reducing the risk of osteoporosis.

- Exercise helps bolster the immune system, which protects against everything from cancer to the common cold.

- Exercise helps keep joints healthy and workable, thus reducing the chances of arthritis.

- Exercise develops the lower back muscles, thus reducing the chances of recurring back pain.

- Exercise makes the brain more alert and accelerates reaction time, reducing risks of driving accidents and accidents around the home.

- Exercise enhances dexterity, which lowers the risks associated with falling and tripping, particularly among the elderly.

- Exercise improves the ability to fall asleep and sleep well.

- Exercise lowers the resting heart rate because the heart becomes stronger due to the increased quantity of blood it pumps per contraction. In fact, the heart of an inactive person beats 30,000 to 50,000 more times each day than someone who exercises regularly. This saves the heart as many as 17 million beats per year!

- Exercise enriches sexual performance by building endurance and flexibility as well as positive body image and self-esteem.

- Because of all of the above, exercise greatly lowers your risk of an early death.

Regardless of your present condition or age, it's never too late or too soon to begin a life of exercise. What can you lose other than those unwanted, unhealthy extra pounds? Okay, so you might miss a few TV shows, but the rewards will more than outweigh the sacrifices. Your health and quality of life will improve, because you'll look better and feel better both mentally and physically.

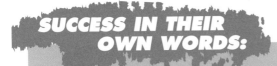

SUCCESS IN THEIR OWN WORDS:

Phil's Story

- Age forty-four, married
- Lost 188 pounds and 11 inches

I hated the way I looked and what I had let myself become. I know my wife wasn't happy with me either. Finally, I became fed up with my weight and state of health. What I did was basic: I changed my way of eating and began exercising. The hardest part was making myself get up and exercise on days I wanted to just lounge around. It was also tough to let go of those comfort foods.

For me, results came fairly quickly, although it took about eighteen months to lose the 188 pounds. Today, I am a different person. People who knew me before and haven't seen me in a couple years don't even recognize who I am. And I'm very active now, whereas before I was a couch potato. I feel like I'm a much better husband and dad to my family.

Phil's Eating Habits:

- I took myself off of sugar and refined flour.

- I eat a lot of vegetables, beans, and grains.

Phil's Exercise Habits:

- Bodyweight resistance training for twenty minutes Mondays, Wednesdays, and Fridays.

- Cardio five times a week for an hour. I have a low-impact elliptical machine that I use while watching TV.

PERSONAL REFLECTION:

How active is your lifestyle? If you exercise, does your exercise come from consistent, regular efforts on your part, or is it hit-and-miss? Do you need to build an exercise program into your life?

YOUR TO DO LIST:

Find an hour a day to devote to exercise. You can break it up into two half-hours if necessary. Can you exercise in the morning before you leave for work? Is there a time in the evening you can squeeze in a workout?

FOR FURTHER STUDY:

www.cooperaerobics.com

The Three Main Forms of Exercise We Need

When you are exercising optimally, you will feel energized, motivated, strong, and have a more positive attitude about life. You'll wonder why you wasted all those years being a couch potato when you could have been an exercise nut.

—SHARI LIEBERMANN

POWER STATEMENT:

For optimum health, our bodies need cardiovascular exercise, strength and resistance training, and flexibility training.

If you are serious about creating a healthy lifestyle and experiencing all the benefits, if you really want to lose weight and keep it off, then you must include exercise. It's not an option. According to a study from the National Weight Control Registry, people who lost at least thirty pounds and kept the weight off burned approximately 2,800 calories a week through planned exercise. When planning your weekly routine, there are three different types of exercise you need to utilize in order to achieve optimum health: cardiovascular or aerobic exercise, strength or resistance training, and flexibility training.

Before we take a look at the three different exercise forms, there are a few common sense warnings to consider.

- Before taking part in any strenuous exercise routine, evaluate yourself first. For some, different forms of physical activity might be unsafe or should only be started after consulting a health professional.

- Drink plenty of water. Dehydration may result from losing too much water from excessive sweating and failing to replace it by drinking it as you work out.

- Do not work out in the extreme heat. In addition to dehydration, heat exhaustion and heatstroke may result from exercising in severe heat and humidity.

- Do not overdo it. Overuse injuries can happen when you overuse certain joints and muscles. In addition, overtraining can cause fatigue and irritability as well.

- Listen to your body. If you have difficulty breathing or experience faintness or pro-longed weakness during or after exercise, consult a healthcare professional.

Cardiovascular/Aerobic Exercise

Some form of steady, uninterrupted cardiovascular or aerobic training for a period of thirty minutes at least three to five times a week is essential. Cardiovascular or aerobic exercise refers to physical exertion that places a healthy strain on the heart, lungs, blood vessels, veins, and capillaries. Just like the muscles, these body parts grow stronger with repeated and augmented use.

One of the main goals of a cardiovascular workout is to increase the heart rate. The result is increased blood circulation, which carries added oxygen to your muscles. This increased blood circulation also aids the body in generating new fat-burning enzymes and is commonly considered the best for controlling weight.

Exercises that apply steady, rhythmic pressure to the chief muscle groups and burn oxygen for extended periods rather than brief bursts are considered cardiovascular or aerobic because they push your heart and lungs to work between 70 and 85 percent of their capacity. The following are what I feel are the three most effective cardiovascular or aerobic exercises.

Power Walking

I used the term "power walking" instead of simply "walking" because the pace makes all the difference. Some people go out for a leisurely stroll and think they are achieving results, but they aren't. Granted, a leisurely stroll is better than being stationary, but the goal of aerobic walking is to get that heart rate up. Walking is an ideal exercise because it builds endurance, burns fat, prevents osteoporosis, diminishes the chances of serious disease, and lifts the emotions.

Begin your regimen with thirty-minute walks, gradually building up to forty-five to sixty minutes over several weeks. As you build muscle and endurance, pick up your pace. Practice your strides until they are smooth and you are breathing rhythmically and moving from your center. Extend your body while you walk, taking long strides with smooth but regular arm motion.

It is the legs that do the walking, but the arms also play a significant role. When walking at a faster pace, try bending your arms at a ninety-degree angle and then swing your fist up to eye level as you bring your arms forward. These exaggerated arm swings promote upper body conditioning. Don't forget to stand straight and use good body posture, focusing on tightening the abdomen muscles and lifting from your lower torso. This strengthens those important but often neglected postural muscles. Leaning forward too much can put unnecessary strain on the lower back.

One drawback to walking is it usually takes longer to achieve optimum results. Ninety minutes of walking equals the same cardio benefits of a thirty-minute run. Walking two miles per hour burns approximately 240 calories per hour; walking four miles per hour burns 440.

However—and it's a big however—a study in the December 2000 *Journal of Sports Medicine and Physical Fitness* found that walking at speeds equal to or greater than five miles an hour (a twelve-minute mile) actually burned more calories than running at the same speeds. If you can do this, the amount of calories you'll burn jumps to 740 per hour! But there is a catch. Walking at this pace is not easy and takes an incredible amount of concentration to keep up the pace. At this speed, it is actually easier for the body to run, which is why you burn more calories walking. If you are going to attempt this kind of power walking, my recommendation is to find a community track, usually at a local high school or middle school, get an inexpensive stopwatch, and time your laps. One lap around a regulation track at five miles an hour would be three minutes.

Also, many communities today have tracks and walking parks. If you don't have access to one of these, you can mark out your own course using your car to measure the distance. My suggestion is you mark out 2.5 miles in one direction. Power walk to that point, and then turn around and power walk back. This would give you five miles and your goal could be to work up to finishing in one hour, which would be five miles an hour. I've done this all over the country when I travel. In addition to a great workout, it's a great way to relax, let your mind unwind, and take in the scenery.

Experienced power walkers increase both their stride length and their step frequency in order to walk faster. To increase the pace, it's not necessary to take giant strides or try to go as fast as a windup toy. You can make a substantial difference in your walking speed by simply taking a few more steps per minute. As you get in better shape, your flexibility of motion will increase, resulting in longer strides, and a faster walking speed will come naturally.

Another advantage to walking over running is that it puts much less stress on the joints, which significantly reduces the likelihood of injury. And because the low impact minimizes the strain on the feet and joints, people are more likely to stick with the activity for the long term.

Also, walking could be divided out over the course of a day relatively easily. For example, a person could do ten minutes in the morning, ten minutes during lunch, and thirty minutes in the evening and have done fifty minutes of walking, although it would be best to eventually be doing the high octane power walk for sixty minutes at one time.

Running

If you can handle the continuous pounding which causes wear and tear on the joints (for some, it's not an issue until they get older), the benefits of running are huge and cannot be overstated. Running is quite possibly is the most effective means to lose weight. And believe it or not, the speed at which you run has little to do with the number of calories you burn. Regardless of how fast you run, you can burn an average of 100 to 150 calories per mile.

Of course, that doesn't mean that running is a magic ticket. It's likely that you may even gain weight in the beginning as the body converts its fat tissue to muscle. So don't get discouraged if progress seems slow at first. Sticking with the program and maintaining consistency are the keys. If you do, you'll eventually see the excess pounds drop off. You'll notice that committed runners seldom have problems with their weight. Another couple of pluses are the health of the heart is vastly increased by the influx of oxygen-rich blood due to better circulation, and running helps flush toxins out of our systems.

The following are some strategies that have proven most successful for runners interested in maximum weight loss. Note that before you begin any type of running program it is critical to purchase regulation running shoes, not walking or tennis shoes. This will create a cushion and help reduce the effects of pounding on your joints.

Set a goal to eventually be running twenty-five to thirty miles per week. It's important to note that it's not necessary to run fast like an Olympian; you simply have to be disciplined enough to put in twenty-five to thirty miles a week of relaxed running.

Run for longer periods at a consistent pace, even if a slow pace. Workouts that last at least sixty minutes or more put you into the fat-burning zone. This is when the body starts to burn stored fats, rather than carbohydrates. But when doing longer workouts like this, do not do them every day, but about three days a week.

Now, I do realize that most people just starting out may not be able to do the above requirements. Don't worry and don't be scared. Start slow, be patient, and enjoy yourself. It's important that you enjoy the running experience in order to stay consistent and become successful. Learning to enjoying running, however, can take time. It's a love that has to be developed, so patience is critical.

You may want to start out by combining walking and running. If so, this is a very effective and popular route to take. The following is a teen-week walk/run plan for beginners to eventually build up to thirty minutes of running per workout. You'll need an inexpensive stop watch to hold in your hands while working out.

Week	Run	Walk	Repeat
1	2 Minutes	3 Minutes	6 Times
2	3 Minutes	2 Minutes	6 Times
3	5 Minutes	2.5 Minutes	4 Times
4	7 Minutes	3 Minutes	3 Times
5	8 Minutes	2 Minutes	3 Times
6	9 Minutes	1 Minute	3 Times
7	9 Minutes	1 Minute	3 Times
8	13 Minutes	2 Minutes	2 Times
9	14 Minutes	1 Minute	2 Times
10	30 Minutes		

Jumping Rope

Jumping rope is another one of the prime cardio-vascular/aerobic workouts for building the heart's endurance and shedding excess pounds. Boxers have known this for years. Jumping rope actually burns about the same amount of calories per hour as power walking five miles an hour or running. Fifteen minutes of jumping rope can burn anywhere from 150 to 200 calories. That's 800 calories in an hour! In addition, it gives an excellent total body workout. And the beautiful thing is; you can do it anywhere, anytime, in front of the TV and regardless of the weather. It's a great workout for the wintertime months and if you are traveling. Many people actually coordinate their jumping with their favorite music, creating a more lively workout.

When you start, you'll want to purchase a quality, heavy, regulation exercise rope, the heavier the better because it makes the rope move more smoothly. As with all the other aerobic exercises, it's important to begin slowly and build up endurance over a period of time. Don't attempt to jump for fifteen consecutive minutes until you've built up your endurance.

Instead, do one-minute intervals, resting at least thirty seconds between jumps. Repeat this for as many minutes as you can. If you are heavier or terribly out of shape, don't get discouraged, just do what you can do and improve a little more each time. As you become more fit, gradually increase the length of your jumping intervals and decrease the length of your rest. Remember, when jumping, regardless of how good you are, it only counts as a rest period if when you stop you don't immediately start back up again. You will gain more coordination the more you practice. Within a matter of weeks you should be able to jump two or more sets of fifteen minutes.

In order to prevent injury, bend your knees when you land and jump on your toes only about an inch off the ground. Be sure to jump on a surface that "gives," such as a wooden floor, carpet, or even grass that is cut short.

Though the above three exercises are the top on my list in the cardio/aerobic category, there are many alternatives that may work for you. Also, because your goal is a lifestyle change, it's important to keep things interesting and fun. So don't be afraid to mix it up a bit. The following are some other great cardio activities that are major calorie burners.

- Bicycling—stationary or outdoors, depending on resistance and speed, bicycling can burn 250 to 500 calories in thirty minutes.

- Swimming—like jumping rope, swimming is a full body exercise and burns approximately 400 calories in thirty minutes.

- Racquetball—intense racquetball burns approximately 400 calories in thirty minutes.

- Cross-country skiing—whether on a machine or on snow, this full body exercise and can burn about 350 calories in thirty minutes.

- Step aerobics—can burn as much as 400

calories in thirty minutes.

- Rollerblading—this is a marvelous way to get low-impact cardio activity. It helps your coordination and burns approximately 300 calories in thirty minutes. More and more middle-aged people are participating in this activity.

- Tennis with a friend or hitting tennis balls alone—depending on your ability and time between sets, burns 200 to 300 calories in thirty minutes.

- Basketball—depending on your intensity, a game of one-on-one can burn up to 400 calories in thirty minutes. If you're on your own, you can shoot hoops and get your own rebounds for a comparable workout.

- Sign up for an aerobics class or take advantage of an aerobics video or DVD. This can be a good way to go because it will help you with consistency and you'll have others there to help you keep up the pace. Plus, you can burn up to 400 calories in a thirty-minute workout.

Whatever you do, be creative. My friend Mr. Paul is seventy-two years old. Looking at him, however, you'd think he's sixty-two, and based on his energy level, you'd think he's twenty-two. The guy never stops. Several times a week you can find him at the local middle school's baseball diamond hitting softballs. He carries a garbage can full of about a hundred balls. Standing on home plate he tosses one up

on Losing Weight

and whacks away, sending softballs like bullets into the outfield. When the garbage can is empty, he goes around and picks up all the balls and then starts over. One day we were talking and he told me it was his goal to hit 10,000 balls in one year! Creativity is one

PRACTICAL TIP #16

Develop a habit of aerobic exercise at least three times a week. Keep it simple—there's no need to sign up for a gym membership or buy expensive home equipment if you have a walking track near your house. And make it fun—burn mix CDs of your favorite workout music, bring friends or dogs along on your walks, or buy your favorite sitcom on DVD to watch while you jump rope or ride a stationary bike.

of the best ways to beat the boredom blues. And everyone knows that time flies when you're having fun.

Strength and Resistance Training

Regardless of your sex or age, and particularly as you grow older, it's imperative that you devote at least fifteen to twenty minutes to strength training two or three times a week. To be at optimal health, you need muscle mass. Why? Because muscle is critical to weight control. You see, muscle is the best calorie-burning tool the body has. Unlike fat, muscle burns calories even when we are resting. In fact, muscle burns calories twenty-four/seven. It makes perfect sense, then, that the more muscle we have, the more calories we burn.

Another important fact to consider is that after the age of twenty a person loses approximately seven percent of their overall muscle mass every decade. Since body weight is more apt to increase over time for most people, most usually do not recognize that they are losing their muscles as they age. Yet between the ages of twenty and seventy, a person can lose 30 to 40 percent of their muscle mass due to muscular degeneration.

The question I want to ask you now is this: What do you think replaces the withered muscle mass? The answer is fat. So just by aging, 30 to 40 percent of your body's muscle will eventually turn to fat. Fat burns much fewer calories than muscle. As I already stated earlier in the book, a single pound of resting muscle burns fifty calories per day compared to a pound of fat that burns a whopping three calories! And if our food intake is not decreased, that will add to even more fat. This causes what many call "creeping obesity." But don't get depressed, because there is hope. This loss of muscle mass can be reversed or significantly reduced in most cases by strength and resistance exercise.

Cardio exercises are not effective at building muscle. This is why those who focus primarily on the aerobic aspect of exercise usually gain back the weight they lose very quickly if they stop their exercise regimen. Because of the lack of muscle mass, their calorie-burning is wholly dependent on what they burn during their cardio workouts. Thus, when they stop, their calorie burning slows way down, and their weight goes up.

The cure for this dilemma is to plan into your routine regular strength and resistance training. It's the only category of exercise that that builds lean muscle and boosts the body's metabolism around the clock. Without fail, those who consistently partake in strength and resistance exercises a few times a week for fifteen to twenty minutes lose their excess weight much more quickly, both men and women alike.

If you are concerned about bulking up and looking too muscular, don't worry. That doesn't have to happen. In order to bulk up, you'd have to consume excess calories and do a completely different type of routine than you'll be doing. To stay lean without looking like Mr. Universe, use lighter weights and do more reps on each set of exercises.

Attending a health club with free weights and machines or having weights at home is one route that works well. Sometimes the more progressive machines in a health club can give you an isolated workout on certain muscle groups. However, if that is not an option, there are several strength and resistance exercises you can do anywhere, anytime, without weights. These are called bodyweight exercises, and the results they can give are profound.

Personally, I prefer the bodyweight exercises over free weights or machines, and many other professionals do as well. You can build muscle mass and reach all the strength resistance requirements through bodyweight workouts. Bodyweight training covers the full range of muscle groups that helps build a much more naturally proportioned look than you get by isolating specific muscles with free weights or machines. It's been well known for decades that gymnasts train almost exclusively using bodyweight exercises, and they are renowned for their extraordinary strength and superiorly sculptured physiques. In addition, for years the military has been using bodyweight exercises along with running and marching to get soldiers in optimal shape.

The following are ten standard bodyweight exercises that are effective in enhancing muscle strength and endurance along with giving the body a firm, muscular tone. Though they seem simple, in reality, bodyweight exercises can be more difficult to perform because a person can't lessen the weight according to their own suitability. Instead, they just have to stay focused and press harder throughout the exercise and build up over time.

When working out, always use slow, controlled movement without jerking. Likewise, take slow, controlled breaths. Never do strength and resistance exercises two days in a row—always skip a day between workouts. Your muscles need time to rebuild, and this rebuilding burns even more calories. Remember, technique is more important than speed. The more slowly you do the exercise, the greater the benefit. If you feel that you are losing technique, slow down and do it right even if you have to do fewer repetitions. Doing one repetition with good form is more effective than doing five repetitions with poor form.

As time passes and you gain strength, your routine will change. Some of the exercises are harder than others. On some, you may only be able to do one rep to start. That's okay. Do that one rep and work your way up. If you are not comfortable doing all the exercises, pick the ones you feel confident with and focus on them at the beginning. You will begin to feel results after only one session of these exercises. Imagine what will happen if you do them consistently over months and years.

> ## PRACTICAL TIP #17
>
> Write out a strength training plan. Pick a few days a week when you can devote fifteen to twenty minutes to strength exercises. Tuesdays might be upper body days, Thursdays might be torso days, and Saturdays might be lower body days.

To help you stay focused, I suggest writing your plan and your exercises on an index card. Also, you may want to have two bathroom towels to use for hand cushions.

Pushups

Hands down, pushups are superior for developing an outstanding upper body—chest, triceps, biceps, and shoulders. Though not essential, I recommend purchasing pushup handles. They are a real asset because they give you a deeper press range, aid with proper form, and make the exercise more comfortable to do. Therefore, you're more likely to do more repetitions. They're inexpensive and can be picked up at most stores that sell sporting goods.

Lie facedown on the floor and place your hands on the floor a little more than shoulder-width apart. Push your body up using your arms while keeping your back straight—it's really important that you don't let your back sag in the middle. Next, lower your body until your chest almost touches the floor. Hold for a one count. Push back up and then repeat.

Do three sets of as many as you can with proper form, resting one minute between sets. With consistency and determination, you can eventually be doing three sets of twenty-five or more. To work different parts of the muscles, I suggest doing a set of wide grips, a set of close grips, and a normal-width set. Also, if you are unable to do straight pushups you may want to start with inclined pushups, by pushing against a table or bench. Or you can do pushups with your knees on the floor. The goal, however, is to wean yourself off of modified pushups and eventually be doing conventional pushups.

Dips Between Chairs

Dips target the upper back, triceps, biceps, shoulders, and midsection. Take two chairs or two tables that are sturdy enough to hold your full body weight and place them shoulder width apart, back to back. Grip each chair and bend your legs at the knees. You may want to wrap towels around where you grip the chairs to form cushions. With your body hanging, steady yourself and dip down to where the upper arms are parallel to the floor and then back up again. Do not lock your elbows. Do three sets of as many as you can, resting one minute between sets.

If you find this too difficult, begin with single chair dips. Place the back of the chair against a wall. Facing out, squat in front of the chair and grip both sides of the chair with your hands, then stretch your legs out in front of you. Now, with your legs and back straight and your stomach tight, dip your body down and back up. Do three sets of as many as you can, resting one minute between sets.

Pull-ups and Chin-ups

Pull-ups target the biceps and abs. This exercise requires either purchasing an inexpensive pull-up bar that can be hung in any doorway or having access to a playground or gym. Start by gripping the bar with your hands shoulder-width apart. With your arms straightened, permit your body to hang from the bar while bending your knees and crossing your feet. Next, pull yourself upward to where your chest almost touches the bar. While you are pulling up, focus on keeping your back straight without curving or swinging. After your chest is up to the bar, lower yourself to the beginning position and repeat.

If you're just starting out, don't be discouraged if you can only do one rep. Just be consistent, improving a little each week. Do three sets of as many as you can, resting one minute between sets.

Chin-ups are a slightly different version of the pull-up that works different parts of your biceps, chest, and back muscles. To perform a chin-up, grasp the bar with a reverse underhanded grip the same distance apart as with pull-ups and follow the same sequence as with pull-ups, only underhanded. Do three sets of as many as you can, resting one minute between sets.

Curls

Purchase inexpensive dumbbells, fifteen to twenty-five pounds, or a twenty-five- to forty-five-pound curl bar. If you can't do that, you can fill two empty gallon milk jugs with water or sand. That will work just fine. Stand up with your back straight and let your arms fall down to your sides.

With dumbbells or jugs in each hand, using only your arms, slowly curl your arms to your chest and back down. The key is going very slowly with your back straight. Don't cheat by swinging. Do three sets of as many as you can, resting one minute between sets.

Crunches

Lie on your back and bend your knees up with your feet flat against the floor. This is your starting position. Place your hands on your ears or the side of your head (not behind your head), or cross your arms over your chest or stretch them out straight. Crunch your torso by lifting your shoulder blades about thirty degrees off the floor, placing all the stress on your abdomen, not your back. Then relax back to the starting position and repeat. If you are stretching your arms out, crunch your torso by touching your fingers to the top of your knees. You should do this exercise without anyone holding your feet down. Do three sets of as many as you can, resting one minute between sets. With time, you can eventually be doing 100 to 500 at a time.

Twisting Crunches

To ensure that your side abdominal muscles are not forgotten, try to include some twisting crunches. Begin in the same start position as you did for regular crunches. Crunch your torso up and twist to the left by angling your right shoulder and right elbow toward your left knee. Then crunch your torso up and twist to the right by angling the left shoulder and left elbow towards the right knee. If you're stretching out your arms, touch the right fingers to the left knee and alternate. Come back through the center and return to start position. Do three sets of as many as you can, resting one minute between sets.

Leg Extensions

Kneel on all fours. Make sure you have plenty of space in front and behind you. Look forward and pull your knee up slowly under the chest, then extend the leg backward, making sure you do not raise the leg higher than your bottom. Lower the leg to the start position and repeat with other leg.

Begin by doing out ten extensions on each leg. Increase gradually over time until you can do twenty-five on each leg.

Squats

Stand with feet apart, hands on hips. Squat until your thighs are parallel to the ground. Do not go beyond this point—you won't gain any advantage by going too far, and you could hurt your knees. As you bend your knees, make sure they keep pointing in the same direction as your toes. Return to the start position and repeat. Do three sets of as many as you can, resting one minute between sets.

Back and Butt Builder

This is a great little exercise for sculpting the behind and strengthening the back. Lie facedown with your feet slightly apart and your arms stretched out in front of you. Keeping your head down and your abdominal muscles tightened, lift one leg and your opposite arm six to twelve inches off the floor. Hold for a one count. Do twenty reps and then switch to your other arm and leg for twenty.

Flexibility Training

The third and final component of a balanced exercise program is flexibility. This is vital because flexibility greatly reduces much of the immobility linked with aging and also averts many joint and muscle troubles that some encounter when they exercise without warming up appropriately.

Being flexible doesn't mean that we need to be as bendable as elastic. What it does mean is keeping our muscles and joints pliable enough to avoid pain and discomfort with regular exercise. The flexibility we're talking about here is the ability to move joints and muscles through their full range of motion. It involves stretching the calves, quadriceps, triceps, groin muscles, and hamstrings.

The basis for proper stretching is in the execution of the exercise. While you are stretching, there should be no pain. If you do experience pain or pulling, you are doing something wrong and should ease up. The more stretching you do, the more you will limber up over time. Remember, small gains over time equal big results.

The following are some flexibility exercises developed by the American Academy of Orthopedic Surgeons. These exercises will also help warm up various parts of your body.

Lower Back

Lie flat on your back facing upwards. Grabbing your knee, bring your right leg to your chest. If possible, keep the back of your head on the ground and try keeping your lower back flat. Hold for fifteen to thirty seconds. Repeat with your left leg.

Hip and Groin

Sitting in the upright position, touch the soles of your feet together, then grab your ankles and pull your legs inward. With arms supplying slight resistance on the inside of legs, slowly push down your knees. Try to touch your nose to your feet. Hold for five seconds and repeat several times.

Knee and Calf

Part 1: Standing facing a wall, chair, or fence, steady yourself and hold the top of your left foot with left hand

and gently pull your heel toward your butt. Hold for fifteen to thirty seconds. Repeat with other leg.

Part 2: Leaning forward on a solid support like a wall, with your forearms and head resting on your hands, bend one leg and place your foot on the ground in front of you, with the other leg straight behind you. Slowly move your hips forward, keeping your lower back flat. Hold for fifteen to thirty seconds. Repeat legs. Don't bounce!

Shoulder

Part 1: In a standing or sitting position, interlace your fingers. With your palms facing upward, push your arms back and up feeling the stretch in your arms and shoulders. Hold for fifteen seconds and repeat.

Part 2: With your arms overhead, hold the elbow of one arm with the hand of your other arm. Gently pull the elbow behind your arm. Do this slowly. Hold for fifteen seconds, then switch arms.

Part 3: Gently pull your elbow across your chest toward your opposite shoulder. Hold for fifteen to thirty seconds, then switch elbows.

Hamstring

Sit down and straighten your left leg. The sole of your right foot should rest next on the inside of your straightened leg. Lean forward and touch the toe of your straightened leg with your fingers. Keep your left foot upright with the ankle and toes relaxed. Hold for fifteen seconds and repeat with right leg.

Toe Raises

This stretch will develop the muscle to prevent shin pain when walking and running. Stand upright with your toes over the edge of a raised surface. Only your heels should be on the edge with your toes extended as far out over the edge as you can. Pull your toes upward towards

PRACTICAL TIP #18

Do flexibility stretches before each workout to keep your muscles and joints limber and able.

your shins as far as you can and hold for a second, feeling the contraction in your shins. Slowly lower your toes to the starting position and repeat. Your body should remain upright. Do ten to fifteen repetitions.

These basic flexibility exercises should do the trick in keeping your joints and muscles limber. Remember, have good form, always stretch slowly without pain, and maintain consistency.

To summarize, no exercise program is complete without cardiovascular exercise, strength and resistance training, and flexibility training. Be consistent with these exercises over time, and I promise you'll see incredible results.

SUCCESS IN THEIR OWN WORDS:

Fred's Story

- Age fifty-two, happily married

- No weight loss, but Phil has maintained an extremely healthy and fit lifestyle. At age fifty-two he is more fit than most twenty-five-year-olds. At six-foot-one, Fred is 185 pounds of lean muscle, with about 5% body fat.

I work out and eat healthy out of necessity—for me, it's all about preventative medicine. I want to be as effective as a can be on the job, with my wife and family, and for God. I enjoy my lifestyle and desire to keep it going as long as I can. With God's help, there's no reason why I can't continue like this through my seventies and beyond.

Fred's Eating Habits:

- For me, the perfect breakfast is a small bowl of oatmeal with maple syrup and half an apple with coconut butter.

- At lunch, I stay away from junk food. I usually eat a turkey sandwich or something similar from a sub shop.

- Every day I take an apple and banana to work with me for snack.

- Each day I carry with me a half-gallon jug of water and drink the whole thing by the end of the day. I do this for reverse osmosis effect.

- For dinner, if we eat meat, it's always pretty lean, and we include a lot of vegetables like spinach, cabbage, peas, and beans. We really like hummus, a type of bean dip.

- Each day, I take a multi-vitamin, a Vitamin B supplement, two magnesium tablets for my heart, one chromium tablet, and one niacin for blood flow.

Fred's Exercise Habits:

- I walk a lot every day. When I get home from work, I walk at least a mile to unwind.

- I work as a landscape engineer at a major university. During work, I intentionally park my vehicle in the far end of parking lots so I have to walk.

- In addition to my walking, three or four times a week, I do thirty to forty-five minutes on the step machine. It's an inexpensive, non-electric one that utilizes shock absorbers. I usually read while I work out.

- At home I do pull-ups, dips, two sets of thirty sit ups, and two sets of thirty pushups.

- At night, before I take my shower, I do thirty to forty leg squats.

> • Before sleep and as soon as I wake up, I do
> a few flexibility exercises.

PERSONAL REFLECTION:

Do you feel prepared to start an exercise program?
What gets in the way of exercise for you? How do you
think your life will improve after you form a habit of
exercise?

✓ YOUR TO DO LIST:

Start small. For the next two weeks, build cardio into
your routine three days a week. During the next two weeks, add a
strength and resistance regimen to your cardio. And be sure to
do your flexibility exercises before each workout.

FOR FURTHER STUDY:

The No Sweat Exercise Plan
—by Harvey B. Simon, M.D.

Fitting It in, Doing It, and Maintaining It

One of the most common reasons people give for not working out is lack of time. But that's not really a legitimate excuse and we can prove it!

—BARBARA HARRIS

POWER STATEMENT:

It's not always easy to find time to exercise, but an exercise habit can be built, even in the busiest schedule.

No doubt, for many people life today is a blur of busyness. I bet I know what you're thinking: Between work, fighting traffic, keeping up with the kids, household chores, running to the bank and grocery store, and meeting the demands put upon us from family and friends, it's hard enough to simply get a good night's sleep, much less do all this fitness stuff—is that about right? For some, finding thirty minutes or an hour each day for exercise seems quite impossible. Yet as out of reach as it may seem, if you really want to, you can make the choice to fit fitness in.

Countless people complain that they don't have enough time to exercise when in reality they don't have energy or the want-to. Don't get me wrong—I understand all too well the demands a busy life can thrust upon you. I have a busy life myself. But the hard truth is, the majority of people, even busy people, who say they can't find the time to work out, will spend an hour a day on the computer surfing the Web and checking email or watching TV. If you believe that you don't have the time, you need to do some rethinking, because you can make it work if you simply make some modifications to your daily routine. All of this may sound somewhat extreme. However, it is critical—and I mean critical—that you fully grasp that if you do not exercise now, you will pay for it later. The statistics prove it.

Unfortunately, this is one area where there is no simple

solution that will produce magical results. But you need not despair. It's not really that difficult to fit exercise into an already crowded lifestyle if you really want to. It can be done. And once you do, you will see your life open up like never before because you'll be more efficient both psychologically and physically. You'll feel better and have more energy to accomplish more. On top of that, working out itself can be fun—and should be. I can't think of any better reasons for modifying your lifestyle than those. Can you?

Here are a few tips to help you make the needed adjustments.

Make a commitment, even if it's a small one, to exercise at least four days a week. The choice to implement a fitness routine into your life is not something to take lightly. Long-term results require being absolutely convinced of the benefits of exercise and of the risks of non-exercise. It's a lifelong commitment of time and effort. To succeed, exercise has to become one of those things that you do without question, just like bathing and brushing your teeth. And now is the time, not tomorrow, not next week. Why would you put off feeling better? That would be crazy. Go ahead make the personal commitment to a healthier lifestyle change and start feeling better today.

Bust the excuses. There are a plethora of excuses you can use for not starting and following through. Each time you make an excuse for not keeping your commitment, bust yourself. This happens by being mentally prepared to deal with your own excuses before they come up. Half the battle is being aware of the excuses that you commonly use. Remember, the hardest part of creating change is getting started— initially and then again each new day. I can tell you from personal experience, the days that I feel the most lethargic and

> **PRACTICAL TIP #19**
>
> Get some accountability. Tell your spouse or a friend about your workout goals, and you'll be more likely to fulfill them.

don't want to exercise are the days I need it the most. Many a day, I have literally forced myself to get with the program, and every time, without fail, after following through I've always been so glad that I did. As you have this same experience time and again, eventually your way of thinking will change and you will view exercise time as a treasured medicine that you can't live without.

Confront the lies. A voice in our head tells us that carving out the time to exercise is impractical, inconvenient, way too time consuming, and we can never do it. Well, it's just not true. People are doing it all the time, all around you. To be optimally healthy, we must confront these lies and change our thinking.

Simplify. There comes a point in every person's life

when they must simplify their lifestyles so they can focus on what's really important. One writer said, "Never let the urgent take the place of the important." We live such urgent lives that we let the really important things in life slip right by. Hans Hauffman wrote, "The ability to simplify means to eliminate the unnecessary, so the necessary can speak." With exercise, the goal is not to cram another activity into your already hectic life, but to arrange your life so you can focus on what's truly important. That will mean learning to say "no" to some demands and people. To be

> ## PRACTICAL TIP #20
>
> Be creative about working exercise into your schedule. Find time to work out during your lunch hour, or work out during your favorite TV show.

successful in one area, sometimes it's necessary to let go of others. I have a friend, for example, who desired to succeed in writing. To reach his goals, he chose to give up his hours on the golf course so he could spend more time writing. He had friends that really wanted him to play, but his dream was to write and he knew it would never come to pass unless he made some radical changes to his lifestyle. So he made a choice and made a change. You can too.

Practice better time management. If you have a hectic lifestyle, the only way to be more productive is to become more organized. In fact, if you desire to be fit physically and mentally, the busier you are, the more organized you need to be. Here are some time management tips for implementing exercise into a busy schedule.

- Set realistic goals for diet and exercise. Be sure to include short-term goals to start with, followed after a while by long-term ones. Write down your goals and post them where you can see them every morning and night.

- Put together an action plan and schedule for fulfilling your goals. Write down your schedule and exercises on an index card and keep it with you. Never assume that you'll just fit exercise in on the spur of the moment. Unless you plan the time to work out, it probably won't happen. There are too many distractions to knock you off course.

- Be flexible. If you miss a workout, don't get discouraged or beat yourself up. Just pick up where you left off next time. Realize that interruptions are a part of life. Remember, a little with consistency goes a long way. After a while, exercise will be a natural part of your lifestyle. Give yourself a few weeks to develop a routine you feel comfortable with.

Obviously, there will be times when you can't squeeze in the time to do your complete workout. In times like these, a short workout can do a world of good. Even though a ten- or fifteen-minute workout will not create major increases in your body's fitness, by at least by staying active you won't lose the progress you had previously made. Plus, if your goal is losing weight, burning a few extra calories never hurts.

Remember, keep moving and you always will. The little things add up. Avoid a sedentary lifestyle at all costs.

I have a friend named Nick. When you meet Nick, you are automatically drawn to his high energy and zest for life. You would never know by just looking at him that Nick is eighty-four years old. The fall during the year I wrote this book, he and his wife drove from Louisiana to New England to see the spectacular foliage. His mind is incredibly sharp. In fact, he teaches a class of over two hundred adults each week and has a national radio show. One day, amazed at his physical condition. I asked him, "What's your secret?"

With a sparkle in his eye, he responded, "Forty years of consistent exercise, running, walking, and staying active." After getting to know him better, I found out that Nick was not just a runner, but he took great concern in taking care of his overall health. It's called preventative medicine. I don't know about you, but that is what I want. I want a rich quality of life now and a richer quality of life later. I don't want to merely grow old, but be effective in my older age. The choices you make today will not only have great effects in the present but will carry on into later years.

I know another person, and I won't mention his name, who is also in his eighties. This person has a great mind and is wonderful human being; however, he never exercised and led a very sedentary lifestyle, choosing to do very little physical activity. Even when he had time off, he never exercised. As he began to progress in his years, he began to have physical problems, particularly stiff muscles. Eventually, his legs and hips stiffened up completely, and today he has to be lifted into a car, lifted in and out of a chair and bed. He has to be helped to stand and can barely walk. The sad thing is that most of this could have been prevented if he would have just kept moving over the years. Even if you can't work out as much as you would like, there are many little things you can do during the day that keep you moving, burning calories, and continuing in a fitness state of mind.

- Instead of riding elevators or escalators, take the stairs. Always!

- At the mall or supermarket, park in the farthest parking spot. Even take a couple extra laps around the market too.

- Exercise while watching TV.

- Instead of going out to dinner, go out and walk or rollerblade or do something fun and physical.

CRASH COURSE on Losing Weight

- When visiting a friend, plan a walk.

- At work, instead of taking coffee breaks, take walk breaks.

- Cut your grass with a push mower. This can be a really effective full body workout. A person could lose a lot of weight during the summer months simply mowing their lawn!

- Do household chores more vigorously. It's amazing how many calories you can burn when you tackle those chores. Vacuuming the floors can burn 175 calories per hour; washing dishes, 120; scrubbing floors, 400; mowing grass, 400; raking leaves, 300; gardening, 400; washing the car, 300. You get the picture. Working around the house, even cleaning, can provide just as effective exercise as working out in a gym.

PRACTICAL TIP #21

Create a workout kit for when you're on the road. Keep a jump rope, stopwatch, and a set of workout clothes in one place so you can pack it easily.

- If you have to travel, plan and pack so that you can continue your exercise practices on the road. Pack a jump rope or stay at a hotel that has fitness facilities. If you're stuck in an airport waiting for a plane, instead of being a couch potato, go for a brisk walk and use your carryon luggage to do curls. It's amazing what you can get done fitness-wise in an airport.

- If possible, walk or bike to work instead of driving. I did this for a couple years when I lived about two miles from my office.

- Do stretching exercises at your desk. This reduces stiffness, muscle tension, and helps with blood circulation which will prepare you for more vigorous activity later on.

- Work out more often for shorter periods. Ten to fifteen minutes in the morning, some crunches at lunch, fifteen or thirty minutes after work.

Barry's On-the-Road Success Story

At age forty-seven, Barry is in the best shape of his life. He can do fifteen chin-ups, fifteen pull-ups, fifty push-ups, and can run a six-minute mile. Yet Barry's life or "at least two-thirds of it," he estimates is spent on the road as a pharmaceutical sales rep. So, how does he stay in such fantastic shape? Here's what he has to say:

- "I do two sets of pushups, crunches, and about fifteen minutes of jump rope before I take a shower and leave my motel room in the morning.

- "Sometimes during the day, usually after lunch if I'm not with a client, I find an appropriate area and go for a brisk thirty-minute walk.

- "When I'm checked back into another motel room in the afternoon, before dinner I do more pushups and crunches, usually in front of the TV watching the news. If the motel has a pool, I may also go for a swim, or if the area is nice, I'll go for a thirty- or forty-minute power walk or run. Occasionally, if the hotel has a fitness area, I'll hop on the treadmill in front of the TV, but most of the time I prefer the outdoors.

- "Then on the days I'm home, I do my regular routine."

Like Barry, you too can find a routine that works for you. And as you begin to change your thinking about exercise and implement into you daily lifestyle cardio, strength, and flexibility, your life will begin to change in ways you never thought possible, not just physically, but psychologically as well. Your whole outlook on life will begin to change.

PERSONAL REFLECTION:

How do you think you might be able to carve out more time for exercise? Is there something you might need to give up in order to devote time to your health?

☑ *YOUR TO DO LIST:*

Invent an office workout for yourself.   Pick a few calisthenics exercises, then schedule them on an index card— "Monday: Pushups. Tuesday: crunches," etc.

FOR FURTHER STUDY:

Kathy Smith Timesaver Workout (video)

CHAPTER 11

Now It's Up to You

The decision to translate desire into action and lose weight must come from within an individual. A spouse or partner can't make you do it, a parent can't make you do it, a friend can't make you do it. Only you can make that decision to lose weight. If you review most of the successes in your life, they occurred because you established a clear goal. More important, you believed that the goal you chose could and would be achieved. The same happens with weight loss.

—JIM KARAS

POWER STATEMENT:

You have the ability to change your body and your life.

Someone once said, "No one can go back and make a brand-new start, but anyone can start from now and make a brand-new ending." Though this is the final chapter in this book, it can be the beginning chapter in your new, healthier, and richer life. What we have come to understand is that health and fitness, looking good and feeling good, is no accident. It takes an adjustment in our thinking and in our daily habits. But these adjustments don't have to be painful or boring. You haven't been given a magic formula that promises overnight success, but proven lifetime principles that when applied assure lasting results through a change in lifestyle.

Hopefully, you've come to the point where your desire to succeed at weight loss and optimal health outweighs your fear of failure. You are ready for change. Now it's up to you to take the initiative and start the journey towards the life that you really want. Don't let the fear of failure hinder you. Remember, when things seem slow or you experience a setback, don't get discouraged—just pick yourself up and keep going. This journey is about progress, not perfection. Success comes through small, consistent changes that add up over the course of time.

You can really do this. Now go for it!

SUCCESS IN THEIR OWN WORDS:

Katie's Story

- Age twenty-one, single, pre-med student
- Lost thirty-five pounds and has maintained it for over a year

I ran track in high school. When I quit, I gained weight. I never thought too much about my eating—I just kind of did what everybody else did. After about a year, I started getting really tired all the time and found myself eating more and more to keep my energy up. I gained more weight, but I never felt full or satisfied. I only craved more and continued to lose energy. When my energy level continued to plummet, I got very depressed as a result of being physically tired all the time. I felt like I was walking around in a body that was not cooperating nor was a part of the real me.

After a while, I knew I didn't want to continue to live this way and decided to make a radical change. Luckily for me, both my father and mother are health advocates and helped put me on the right course. Now, after losing thirty-five pounds and keeping it off, I feel the exact opposite as

I did before. I have loads of energy and can't wait to do my exercises. If I miss one of my running sessions, I feel like I'm missing out on a part of my life.

Katie's Eating Habits:

- I'm constantly paying attention to what I eat.

- I cut way down on the amount of pasta, because it was a bad thing for my body. I used to eat a lot of pizza, and I cut way down on that because it has virtually no nutrients. You have to eat so much of it to feel full.

- I stopped eating out so much. When I do eat out I eat better stuff, things with vegetables and nuts.

- I don't eat as much now, but I let myself savor and taste every bite.

- Being a pre-med student helped me to understand food better.

- One food I really found satisfying and healthy is grains, particularly organic whole-grain cereals like puffed rice and muesli. They're tasty, fun to eat, and good for a quick snack.

- I make sure I get enough protein in my daily diet and load up on vegetables, with very little red meat.

- I eat fish a lot, particularly salmon and tuna.

- I still eat a little bit of everything, even fast food, but I eat much smaller amounts. The truth is, when I eat right, I don't have much time to eat that kind of food.

- I try to drink plenty of water. My biochemistry professor said, "The more uric acid you exert, the longer you live."

Katie's Exercise Habits:

- Walk/run four miles three or four times a week

- Crunches, leg raises, shoulder shrugs with dumbbells, and squats three times a week

PERSONAL REFLECTION:

Do you feel ready for a change? Are you optimistic about success? What setbacks do you think you'll encounter along the way? How do you plan to overcome them?

 ## YOUR TO DO LIST:

Make a six-week commitment to your new exercise and eating routine. Write it out. At the end of six weeks, take a minute to evaluate. How do you feel? Are you seeing results?

FOR FURTHER STUDY:

Your Health . . . Your Choice
—by Dr. M. Ted Morter, Jr., M.A.

Six Weeks to a Healthier Lifestyle

Here's a breakdown of some of the principles we've discussed in this book. Build these habits into your life one at a time to make over your lifestyle—and your body.

Week One:

This is water week. Experiment to find the best, most convenient way for you to drink plenty of water—keep bottles of water in the fridge, or buy a large bottle of water to carry and refill throughout the day. Now's as good a time as any to cut out soda.

Week Two:

Get in the habit of eating a healthy breakfast each morning, starting this week. Think nutrient-rich, calorie light foods—oatmeal, cereal, and fruit, and be sure to include a little protein. Keep drinking water!

Week Three and Four:

Start building your exercise routine this week: Set a goal to do four days of cardio for the next two weeks. See Chapter 9 for information on getting started.

Week Four:

This week, look for ways to cut 250 calories from your daily intake. Fried foods are a prime source of calories. Eat smaller meals and tide yourself over with healthy midmorning and afternoon snacks.

Week Five and Six:

Now that the exercise ball is rolling, get into the habit of doing strength and flexibility exercises a few days a week for the next two weeks. Find a time that works for you, and spread your exercises out throughout the week as needed.

Your eating and exercise habits took years to build, and building new ones won't happen overnight. Don't beat yourself up for setbacks, and reward yourself for successes. As you slowly improve your lifestyle, it's only a matter of time before you start shedding the weight.

PART III

21 DAYS OF INSPIRATION

DAY **1**

Everything is created twice— first mentally, then physically.
—GREG ANDERSON

*If you've sat down to write out
your weight-loss goal,
be encouraged:
Writing out your goals
forces you to visualize them,
which is the first and most
important step to
a healthier, slimmer you.*

DAY

He had the deed half done, who has made a beginning

—HORACE

*Thought for the day:
Everyone who has
ever lost weight
has begun exactly the way
you're beginning,
with small changes.
Even that Jared guy.*

DAY

Know what you want to do, hold the thought firmly, and do every day what should be done, and every sunset will see you that much nearer the goal.
—ELBERT HUBBARD

If you're wondering if exercise is really worth the effort, remember that studies show that physical activity helps preserve lean body mass while you're losing weight— meaning that the weight you lose won't be muscle, which will help ensure that you keep the weight off and look great doing it.

DAY

To go fast, row slowly.
—NORMAN VINCENT PEALE

*If you struggle
to form lasting habits
and aren't losing weight as
quickly as you'd like,
don't panic.
If you form habits slowly,
they're more likely to stick.
And if you lose weight slowly,
it's more likely to be
the result of healthy habits—and
therefore more likely to be a
permanent weight loss.*

DAY **5**

The beginning is the most important part of the work.
—PLATO

One of the hardest things
about getting started with
an exercise program is showing up
at the gym with all those
svelte workout pros.
Remember that we all begin
where we are.
Besides, you don't look out of shape,
you look like the kind of person
who's courageous enough
to make changes. If it helps, work out
with an encouraging friend.

DAY

Reality check: you can never, ever, use weight loss to solve problems that are not related to your weight. At your goal weight or not, you still have to live with yourself and deal with your problems. You will still have the same husband, the same job, the same kids, and the same life. Losing weight is not a cure for life.

—PHILLIP C. MCGRAW

If you're putting too much pressure on yourself to get the weight off, ease up. Yes, losing weight is very important to your health, but understand that you are more than your weight and that losing weight won't solve your problems. The good news is that exercise and healthy eating will help you better cope with the stress of life.

DAY

The whole idea of motivation is a trap. Forget motivation. Just do it. Exercise, lose weight, test your blood sugar, or whatever. Do it without motivation. And then, guess what? After you start doing the thing, that's when the motivation comes and makes it easy for you to keep on doing it.

—JOHN C. MAXWELL

Sure, being and staying motivated is important. Getting your mind engaged is essential. But at some point, it's time to do something. You're already in the game by making a few small changes—some findings report that simply eating breakfast can increase your metabolic rate by 25%.

DAY

There is no chance,
no destiny, no fate,
that can circumvent or
hinder or control the
firm resolve of a
determined soul.

—ELLA WHEELER WILCOX

*It's been done: Lots of people have
lost upwards of 200 pounds
by committing to change.
What most success stories seem to have
in common is a rock-bottom experience
that led to a steeled determination
to lose weight. If you're convinced
you need to change your life and are
determined to do so, you can
overcome years of bad habits.*

DAY

You are never too old to be what you might have been.
—GEORGE ELIOT

You're never too old—or even too uncoordinated—to become an athlete. Plenty of fiftysomethings and non-athletes have grown to love exercise and lead an active lifestyle. You may not finish on the medal stand in a 5K race, but you can become fit, healthy, and more agile than you ever thought possible.

DAY

The good Lord gave you a body that can stand most anything. It's your mind you have to convince.

—VINCE LOMBARDI

One of the best ways to keep yourself motivated is to get support—in fact, some health experts would say that dramatic weight loss is impossible to achieve without emotional support. Join with others in your efforts to get healthier, and have people on hand to call when you're tempted to "slip."

DAY

The higher your energy level, the more efficient your body. The more efficient your body, the better you feel and the more you will use your talent to produce outstanding results.

—ANTHONY ROBBINS

Some research suggests that exercise improves brain function, possibly making it more able to process information. So by exercising, you're not just improving your body— you're turning yourself into an effective, efficient, well-oiled machine. And that's worth a workout even if you don't lose an ounce.

DAY

The man who can drive himself further once the effort gets painful is the man who will win.

—ROGER BANNISTER

*Sometimes it takes a while
to lose any weight at all, and
sometimes the body seems stuck
after just losing a few pounds.
But don't give up: Exercising and
watching your calorie intake is only
making you healthier. Plus, some
studies show that a slimming hormone
"kicks in" once a little body fat is shed,
making weight loss faster and easier.*

DAY

Put your heart into everything you do. A lukewarm effort produces mediocre results. Pour on the passion, and experience intense success in all your achievements.

—TAVIS SMILEY

Some research suggests that music can alter our moods, reduce pain, improve focus—and even aid weight loss. Gather some CDs that make you happy, and you may be well on your way to losing a few more pounds.

DAY

To keep progressing, you must learn, commit, and do—learn, commit, and do—and learn, commit and do all over again.

—STEPHEN R. COVEY

*Keep looking for tricks and tools
to help you eat healthy
and keep up your workout routine.
Nuts and peanut butter, for example,
are a great snack—they're tasty
and make you feel full,
and may even assist weight loss.*

DAY

In taking care of the body, you take better care of the spirit.

—MARIANNE WILLIAMSON

*When you eat better, you feel better—
when your body works better,
you feel calmer and more content.
So keep stocking up on healthy foods.
Some dietitians recommend filling
half your dinner plate with vegetables,
then dividing the other half equally
between protein and starch—a great
way to load up on
body-friendly fiber and vitamins.*

DAY

You are the only person who has control over your eating habits. You can always resist something if you choose to.

—LOUISE L. HAY

*No one said discipline was easy,
only that it was worth it.
Be creative. If you have trouble
putting the brakes on, try brushing
your teeth or popping a breath mint
after you're done eating,
or put your fork down
between bites to slow you down.*

DAY

Give yourself rewards for getting through various stages of a project. Treat yourself to a movie, call a friend, or go for a walk.

—JULIE MORGENSTERN

If your eating and exercise program has no room for fun, chances are good that you won't stick with it. Make exercise fun by getting friends and family members in on the act. Reward yourself for a week of good eating with a smoothie or dessert, and find good foods you love to eat. The whole point of losing weight is to make life richer and more enjoyable, not bland and regimented.

DAY

How long should you try? Until.

—JIM ROHN

If you're stuck looking for ways to cut calories, take a look at your routines. If you have a coffee drink full of sugar and milk or cream on the way to work each morning, that may be a high-calorie expenditure you can avoid. Try switching your beverage to tea with honey. Any time you cut calories, you're that much closer to reaching your ideal weight.

DAY

Take care of your body. It's the only place you have to live.
—JIM ROHN

*Weighing in can be demotivating—
it can make you feel like
your efforts are going nowhere,
when in reality you're reaping health
benefits you may not see right away.
You might consider doing away
with home weigh-ins altogether, opting
not to look at the numbers when you
weigh in at the doctor's office.*

DAY

Perseverance is not a long race; it is many short races one after the other.

—WALTER ELLIOT

Next time you feel hungry,
give yourself fifteen minutes.
This will help you determine
if your hunger is physical hunger
or just a passing craving.
Hang in there!
Retraining your body and mind
when it comes to eating isn't easy,
but it's well worth the effort.

DAY

The desire accomplished is sweet to the soul.
—*KING SOLOMON*

*Just think: You're twenty-one
days in to a new life
and a new body.
Next time you're tempted
to give up, remember how much
you'll feel and look better
if you stick with
your new lifestyle.*

PART IV

7-DAY PERSONAL JOURNAL

Keeping a food and exercise journal is a great way to help you take stock of how you're eating, take note of weak moments, and make conscientious decisions. Following is a sample journal. Stick with it for seven days, then stop to evaluate what you're eating and what you might need to change.

SUNDAY

Breakfast:
_____
_____
_____
_____

Snack:
_____
_____
_____
_____

Lunch:
_____
_____
_____
_____

Snack:
_____
_____
_____
_____

Dinner:
_____
_____
_____
_____

Physical Activity:
_____
_____
_____
_____

MONDAY

Breakfast:
_____
_____
_____
_____

Snack:
_____
_____
_____
_____

Lunch:
_____
_____
_____
_____

Snack:
_____
_____
_____
_____

Dinner:
_____
_____
_____
_____

Physical Activity:
_____
_____
_____
_____

TUESDAY

Breakfast:
_____
_____
_____
_____

Snack:
_____
_____
_____
_____

Lunch:
_____
_____
_____
_____

Snack:
_____
_____
_____
_____

Dinner:
_____
_____
_____
_____

Physical Activity:
_____
_____
_____

WEDNESDAY

Breakfast:

Snack:

Lunch:

Snack:

Dinner:

Physical Activity:

THURSDAY

Breakfast:
_____
_____
_____
_____

Snack:
_____
_____
_____
_____

Lunch:
_____
_____
_____
_____

Snack:
_____
_____
_____
_____

Dinner:
_____
_____
_____
_____

Physical Activity:
_____
_____
_____
_____

FRIDAY

Breakfast:
_____
_____
_____
_____

Snack:
_____
_____
_____
_____

Lunch:
_____
_____
_____
_____

Snack:
_____
_____
_____
_____

Dinner:
_____
_____
_____
_____

Physical Activity:
_____
_____
_____
_____

SATURDAY

Breakfast:

_____
_____
_____
_____

Snack:

_____
_____
_____
_____

Lunch:

_____
_____
_____
_____

Snack:

_____
_____
_____
_____

Dinner:

_____
_____
_____
_____

Physical Activity:

_____
_____
_____
_____

NOTES

Chapter 2

[1] Jim Karas, *Flip the Switch* (New York, NY: Random House, 2002), 106-109

Chapter 6

[1] "Position of The American Dietetic Association: Vitamin and Mineral Supplementation," www.eatright.org/asupple

BIBLIOGRAPHY

Bauman, Alisa, and Beth Moxey Eck, "The Walk/Run Way to Weight Loss." Web article: www.runnersworld.com/article/0,5033,s6-51-183-0-1693,00.html.

Blonz, Ed, *Power Nutrition.* New York: Signet, 1998.

Brock, Rovenia M., Ph.D., *Dr. Ro's Ten Secrets to Livin' Healthy.* New York: Bantam, 2004.

Broer, Ted, *Maximum Energy.* Lake Mary, FL: Siloam Press, 1999.

Ferguson, James M., M.D., *Habits Not Diets.* Palo Alto, CA: Bull Publishing Company, 1988.

Galloway, Jeff, *Galloway's Book on Running.* Bolinas, CA: Shelter Publications, 1984.

Golan, Ralph, M.D., *Optimal Wellness.* New York: Ballantine Books, 1995.

Harris, Barbara, *Shape of Your Life.* Carlsbad, CA: Hay House, Inc. 2003.

Jordan, Peg, *The Fitness Instinct.* Emmaus, PA: Rodale Press, Inc., 1999.

Karas, Jim, *Flip the Switch.* New York: Random House, 2002.

Koenig, Larry, *The Smart Discipline Plan for Permanent Weight Loss.* Baton Rouge: Larry Koenig and Associates, LLC, 2000.

Levine, Suzanne, D.P.M., *Walk It OFF!* New York: Penguin Books USA, Inc., 1990.

Liebermann, Shari, Ph.D., CNS, FACN, *Dare to Lose.* New York: Penguin Putnam, 2002.

McGraw, Phil, *The Ultimate Weight Solution.* New York: Simon & Schuster, Inc., 2003.

Meyer, Joyce, *Look Great Feel Better: Twelve Keys to Enjoying a Healthy Life Now.* New York: Warner, 2006.

Morter, Ted, Jr., M.A., *Your Health ... Your Choice.* Hollywood, FL:

Lifetime Books, Inc., 1997.

Null, Gary, *Gary Null's Ultimate Anti-Aging Program.* New York: Kensington Publishing Corp, 1999.

Powter, Susan, *Stop the Insanity.* New York: Simon & Schuster, 1993.

Ralston, Jeannie, *Walking for the Health of It.* Glenview, IL: AARP Publishing, 1986.

Rodgers, Bill, *Lifetime Running Plan.* New York: Harper Collins, 1996.

Sheats, Cliff, *Lean Bodies.* Fort Worth, TX: The Summit Group, 1992.

Shimer, Porter, *Too Busy to Exercise.* Pownal, VT: Storey Communications, Inc. 1996.

U.S. Department of Health and Human Services. *Physical Activity and Health: A Report of the Surgeon General.* Atlanta, GA: U.S. Department of Health and Human Services, Centers for Disease Control and Prevention, National Center for Chronic Disease Prevention and Health Promotion, 1996.

Foods That Harm, Foods That Heal (Pleasantville, NY: Reader's Digest Association, 1996).

Greiwe JS, Kohrt WM. *Energy Expenditure During Walking and Jogging.* (Journal of Sports Medicine and Physical Fitness, 2000).

Centers for Disease Control and Prevention *Increasing Physical Activity: A Report on the Recommendations of the Task Force on Community Prevention Services,* 2001.

U.S. Department of Health and Human Services, "Physical Activity Fundamental to Preventing Disease." Web article: www.aspe.hhs.gov/health/reports/physicalactivity.com.

Walking vs Running Study, *Journal of Sports Medicine and Physical Fitness,* December, 2000.